A Body of Worship

Thank you Lauren!
I hope this book is
a blessing to you!

A Body of Worship

A Fitness Devotional To Help You
Serve God Longer & Serve God Stronger

Kara Bruegger

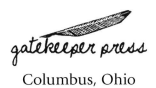
gatekeeper press

Columbus, Ohio

A Body of Worship: A Fitness Devotional To Help You Serve God Longer & Serve God Stronger

Published by Gatekeeper Press
2167 Stringtown Rd, Suite 109
Columbus, OH 43123-2989
www.GatekeeperPress.com

The cover design, interior formatting, typesetting, and editorial work for this book are entirely the product of the author. Gatekeeper Press did not participate in and is not responsible for any aspect of these elements.

Library of Congress Control Number: 2020941164

ISBN (paperback): 9781662901256
eISBN: 9781662901263

In loving memory of my sister,
Kristy Wasicek.
1980-2014

A special thanks to my loving & supportive husband, children, and parents.
Without you guys, none of this would be possible.

Contents

Introduction

Like most people, I have struggled. I have struggled emotionally, spiritually, and physically. But during each challenging season of life, I constantly try to learn from the situation and look for God's work through the storms. Trying to discover God's plan for my life during the twists and turns of life has led me to an amazing passion. It has developed over time, and I'm confident it will continue to mature as I do. But God has led me here and I'm so grateful for it. My life's passion is to encourage others to live a healthy and fulfilled lifestyle. It shouldn't be just another chore on our to-do list. Exercise is a privilege that many people don't have as a physical option. Although, some bodies may have physical limitations, they are capable of so much. After the sudden death of my older sister I became determined to inspire people to exercise and find joy in it.

That's how my journey started. My sister, Kristy, passed away from a brain aneurism at the age of 33. I have always been an active person, but my sister was quite the opposite. So, after her death, I couldn't help but to think, "What if I'd encouraged her to be active with me? Would she still be alive?" Only God knows the answer to that, but I couldn't bear the thought of allowing anyone else to lose a loved one that maybe just needed some encouragement. I became a Mat Pilates instructor and thrived on creating a non-threatening and fun environment.

During my years in front of fitness classes, under fluorescent lighting, in front of huge mirrors, and in skin tight clothing, I started to pick myself apart. I had an idea of what a fitness instructor should look like and I was hard on myself in the areas where I fell short. On top of that, I learned I have an autoimmune disease which makes losing weight and having excess energy increasingly difficult.

It was an awful combination: vanity and fatigue! I wanted to look a certain way but didn't have the energy to put in all that effort. And have I mentioned I'm a notorious emotional eater? If you have bad news for me, you might as well bring a hamburger with you as you break it to me. I was in a losing battle every day and it was exhausting. I couldn't help but think, "There has to be more than this!"

While participating in a diet/reading plan at church, I learned the practice of dedicating my health to God. What an incredible concept! During the ten-day detox that this particular plan called for, I needed prayer and a lot of it. God became a mighty helper in yet another way in my life. I dedicated the next ten days of my life to God and the outcome was more than I could have imagined- more than I could have done on my own.

I would love to say that after the detox session I was a brand-new woman and never faltered with the eating plan that my autoimmune disease requires, but that is far from the truth. The saying "can't teach an old dog new tricks" hit home for me in the time following my successful detox. I fell off the "devote your eating habits to the Lord" wagon for about a year until my doctor suggested a vegan diet for my health. I laughed off the doctor's suggestion for a while until my health started to take a quick decline. If I ever needed Jesus, that was the time. I rocked the vegan diet for a whole three months (sarcasm intended) and felt the physical benefits, but when the holidays came around, veganism was pushed to the back burner. No way Thanksgiving was going to happen without my mom's turkey and cornbread stuffing. What was intended to be a day-long break ended up lasting a whole year. Oops!

Fast-forward through a year of continued health and emotional struggles to the epiphany that reminded me of the diet/reading plan that had taken place such a long time before. How could I experience such a tremendous experience of health and spiritual growth only to do a complete 180 degrees in the time afterwards? The answer is easy, I am a human living for human satisfaction. At that moment I decided to dedicate my health, my eating, my exercise, and my job as a fitness instructor to the Lord. It did not happen overnight. The Lord was patient with me and took His time in teaching me the discipline of having *A Body of Worship*. This book is intended to share with you what the Lord so generously shared with me. Who am I to keep this to myself? It's life changing stuff!

If you are like me (and you probably are because we're both fallen humans with human desires), then I pray that this book holds some answers that you have been searching for. If trying to look a certain way or reaching a certain earthly goal is leaving you feeling anything less than fulfilled, then this book is for you. The freedom that comes from devoting your health, eating habits, and fitness routines as worship is life-altering.

In this book, you will discover what the Bible says about our bodies, the importance of self-control and self-discipline, renewal, and how God will support you during this new adventure. This month-long program is divided into four weeks. Each week we will dive deep into one of the topics listed above. Six days of the week will have guided devotionals followed by safe, non-impact exercise routines. And just like in the Bible, on the seventh day, we will rest.

I pray for you, dear reader. I pray for your devotion to this program and for an open heart that will allow God's word to penetrate and reside. Guard yourself, as I must do as well, from vanity and selfish ambitions. Going forward, it is not about defining our abs or about how well our jeans fit - although that will happen also - but it is all about giving glory to God and devoting our body and all that it can do to the Lord. God has a plan for you and me, and we must be ready to put our "yes" on the altar when the time comes. Let's not limit our abilities due to general unhealthiness. By being healthy, we will be ready to carry out God's will for our lives.

The true takeaway from this book that I hope you receive is that our bodies are not our own. They are the dwelling place of the Holy Spirit who abides in every believer. We are to take care of it- not for our own pride or vanities but out of caring for the Spirit's temple. When we change our focus from having to be super fit or looking a certain way to understanding that we need to be good stewards of our bodies, the pressure is off of us and the glory goes to God. Our culture needs a shift in body image. In a world of selfies and over-inundated social media, it is easy to set our goals to a certain look or body type. We must remember that "healthy" looks different on every body. We strive to be healthier so we may serve our God better and serve Him longer.

Notes About the Fitness Routines

The exercises in this program are all non-impact motions, meanings they are safe on joints. People of all fitness levels will be able to complete the daily series. Exercise modifications (making it easier) and progressions (adding challenge) will be provided when available, so you are able to make the exercise your own.

If you have any injuries or are pregnant, please obtain a doctor's clearance before starting this or any other fitness regimen.

One series per week will call for hand weights. I suggest having two sets of different poundage available. That way you can move throughout the weights as you see fit for you. Larger muscles (i.e. biceps and trapezoids) can handle the heavier weights and the smaller muscles (i.e. triceps and shoulders) may require switching to the lighter set. Remember, it is more effective to have less weight and proper form than to be struggling to keep the form and just throwing heavy weights around. During this program, you will learn to honor your body for what it can do; even in its limitations. When your body is approaching its limit, honor your body by opting for the lighter weights so you can complete the series more effectively. If you do not own hand weights and do not have access to any, canned goods are a good substitute. Also, due to the repetitive nature of the arm series, using no weights at all may be effective as well.

The exercises are interchangeable. If you notice your body does not perform a certain exercise well, that's ok. Remember we are honoring God with our bodies. Not in just what it is able to do but also in abiding in its limitations. Simply, exchange the exercise with another that better suits your abilities.

The symbol, *, will point out what I call "Mile Markers". These are goals for each exercise that we want to try and reach before the end of the program. For example, if the goal is to complete a sixty-second plank, it will be notated by the * symbol. If you are not able to reach the "Mile Marker" during that day's exercise routine, don't be discouraged. That can be a new goal of yours. How exciting! "Mile Markers" will be repeated throughout the month so you can take note of your improvements.

During exercise, it is easy to forget to breath. Our body needs oxygen during exercises to help the recovery time of the growing muscles. Here's a good rule to follow: during the exertion of energy is when you exhale. So, when you feel yourself grunting, that is the proper time to exhale. You want to feel your ribcage move during the breath. The ribs expand on the inhale and they come back in on the exhale.

Before every routine we need to warm up our bodies to avoid injury, especially if it is first thing in the morning or if we've been sitting down for a while. The warmup will be the same every morning. Please refer to the guide below until you have the time to remember the warmup for yourself. The same pertains to the cool down. We need to stretch and give our muscles plenty of oxygen to help our bodies as they recover from the exercises. Please refer to the guide below until you have remembered it over time.

Warm Up

Take a moment before beginning the warm up to pray this simple prayer:

"Lord, I pray that you bless this time. I pray that you are in the center of my efforts and ambitions. I dedicate this time and energy to you. Amen."

FULL BODY STRETCH:

1. Stand with your feet together. Inhale, bring your arms to the ceiling and lift your head.
2. As you exhale, slowly forward fold to your lowest point.
3. Inhale, slightly bend your knees and slowly roll up through the spine. Feel each vertebra stack on top of each other. Bring your arms to the ceiling and look up.
4. Exhale, forward fold. This time, bend your legs into a tuck position allowing your heels to leave the floor.
5. Inhale, place heels back on the floor and slowly begin to roll up. Keep hands by your sides.
6. Repeat 2-3 times.

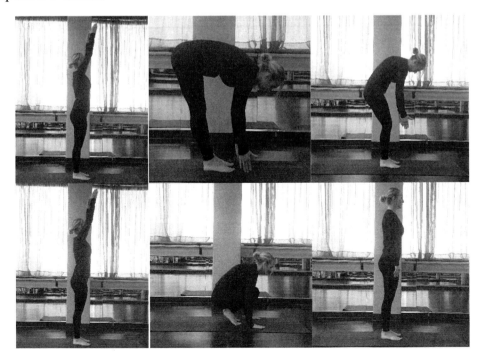

SQUAT & HAMSTRING STRETCH:

1. Open your legs wider than your hips. Toes pointing front. Bend your knees to your lowest comfortable position. Hinge forward from the hips and engage your abdominals. Press your hands together and lift your elbows.
2. While not moving the upper body, extend the knees to stretch the back of the thigh.
3. Return to your squat position.
4. Repeat stretch 4 times.

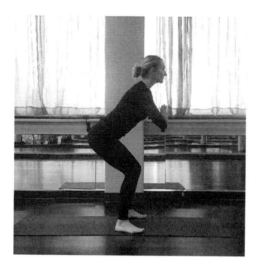

SIDE TWISTS:

1. Keep your legs wider than your hips, turn out from the hips. Toes will be pointing to the diagonal. Bend at the knees.
2. Lengthen your spine to the ceiling and bring your arms to a 90-degree angle in front of the shoulders.
3. Slowly twist to the right, come center, then twist to the left. Repeat 4 times on each side.

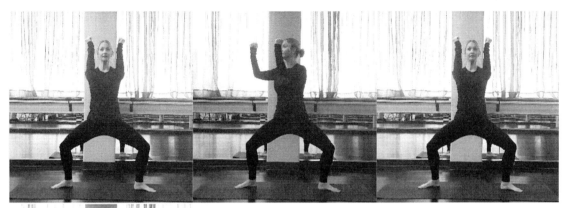

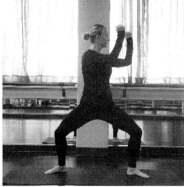

SIDE BENDS:

1. Keep legs in same turned out position and extend the arms to the sides straight from the shoulders.
2. Take the right arm up and over to the left. Hold for 5-10 seconds. Lift to return the arm to shoulder height.
3. Repeat on left side.
4. Repeat on both sides 2-3 times.

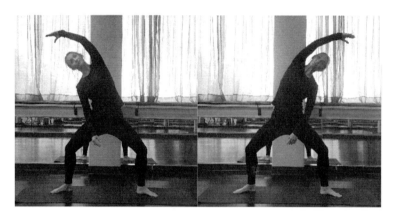

C-CURVE STRETCH:

1. Stand with legs wide and arms out to the sides at shoulder height.
2. Drop the head, curve the back, and roll the hips forward. Reach the arms long in front to stretch out your upper back. Hold for 3 seconds.
3. Lift head to ceiling, press the chest forward, roll the hips away from the ribs. Reach arms behind to stretch the chest. Hold for 3 seconds.
4. Repeat series 3 times.

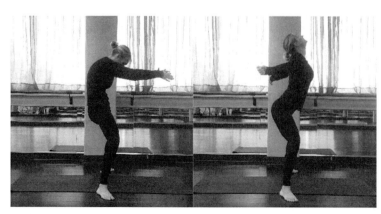

Cool Down

Before your cool down, spend a moment in prayer:

"Lord, I thank you for what my body was able to accomplish during this time. I pray, as I go about my day, that my focus remains on you. Please give me strength, patience, and grace as I work towards having A Body of Worship. Amen."

FULL BODY RELAXATION:

1. Lay on your back with your arms by your sides. Close your eyes.
2. Focus on your breath. Feel the ribcage expand with every inhale and come back in on the exhale.
3. Allow your body to relax. Start by focusing on all of the muscles in your face. Allow the forehead to smooth and your jaw to unclenched.
4. Feel your head getting heavier into the floor, your shoulder blades, your elbows, and your hands all relax and lower deeper into the floor.
5. Allow the same to happen with your tailbone, the back of your calves, and lastly, your heels.
6. Stay here for a moment to focus on what all you accomplished today.
7. When you're ready, wiggle your toes and fingers. Hug your knees to your chest and rock side to side.

LEG STRETCH:

1. Bring your right leg up and point your toes to the ceiling. Grab behind your thigh or calf (never behind your knee), and if you'd like a deeper stretch, gently pull your leg closer towards your chest.
2. Flex your foot, then point your toes. Roll your ankle slowly in both directions.
3. Place your left hand on the outside of the right thigh. Allow the right leg to gently fall across the body to your left. If the stretch is too deep, bend the right knee.
4. Keep both shoulder blades on the floor and allow your head to gently fall to the right to complete the spinal twist.
5. Hold for 8-15 seconds and repeat on the left leg.

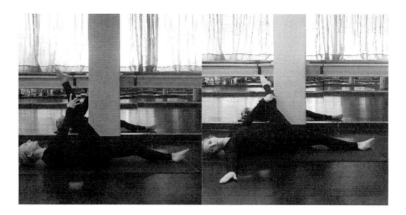

CHILD'S POSE:

1. Slowly prop yourself up from the floor. Sit on your knees with your legs wider than your hips and your feet under your tailbone.
2. Inhale, reach up.
3. Exhale, forward fold to your lowest point.
4. Allow your forehead to rest on the floor and roll your hips back and up to stretch the lower back.
5. Stay in Child's Pose until you feel completely stretched then slowly roll up.

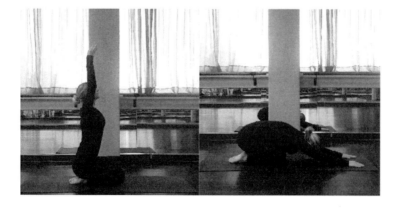

WEEK ONE

A Body of Worship is holy and a living sacrifice.

Week One – Day One

1 Corinthians 3:16-17

> *"Don't you know that you yourselves are God's temple and that God's Spirit dwells in your midst? If anyone destroys God's temple, God will destroy that person; for God's temple is sacred, and you together are that temple."*

Imagine walking past your local church and witnessing someone defacing the building with graffiti. What would you do? I don't think anyone could move about their day without being deeply disturbed by seeing such a blatant act of disrespect towards the house of God.

The Bible tells us that when we accept Jesus Christ as our savior, the Holy Spirit moves into our hearts so He can begin his work in us. Our bodies become holy temples. Let that sink in for a moment. That alone should transform the way we look at ourselves. When we honor our bodies by taking proper care of them, we are honoring God by caring for His habitation.

Let's go back to the illustration of those hooligans defiling the church building. It would be truly upsetting to watch such an act. Many of us would physically do something to stop it and even help restore it to its original beauty. Yet somehow, our culture of instant gratification and increased vanity has led us astray from viewing our bodies as we are meant to- a temple belonging to God himself. A world of busy schedules and convenience foods has blinded us from the fact that we are, metaphorically, painting graffiti on our holy temples with some of the decisions we make. Take your finger off of the spray paint canister and set it down. It is time to restore your temple to its original beauty!

We need to remove the blind folds that we have been tricked into wearing. I want you to hear this… You are special! Your body is special! Your body is sacred! Realize that everything you choose to do with your body has a consequence- either negative or positive. Are you vandalizing your sacred place or are you enhancing its beauty? We are in charge of managing this gift God has given to us- our bodies; the place where the Holy Spirit himself resides in all believers.

Before we move on to the exercise portion for today, please take a moment to re-read the Bible verse above. As you move about the exercises, allow your mind to focus on the passage. What are some things you're currently doing that is vandalizing your temple? In what ways are you nurturing it?

DAY ONE FITNESS ROUTINE

Please refer to the warm up on Page xv to prepare your body for today's exercise routine.

LUNGES:

1. Standing with your head over your shoulders, your shoulders over your hips, and your hips over your ankles, place your hands on your hips.
2. Engage the abdominal muscles by hugging them around your spine- feeling it in the front, back and sides.
3. Place an imaginary string on top of your head and allow it to pull you taller towards the ceiling.
4. Step back with the right leg, placing the ball of your foot on the floor (heel is lifted).
   Modification: For help with balance, place a chair to the side of you and hold a lightly.
   Progression: Lift front heel as well.
5. Bending both knees, bring the right knee closer towards the floor.
6. Hold this lunge position.
   Progression: Attempt to pulse a little lower 5-10 times.
7. Step together.
8. Repeat on the left side. Repeat 10-15 times.

   Rest if needed and repeat the series 2-3 times.

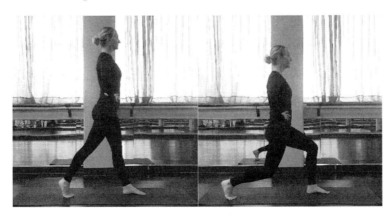

Lunge Notes:

-Be cautious not to hinge forward from the waste. Keep shoulders over hips throughout the series.

-As you step back, allow the front leg to shift back at the hip as well. When you bend into your lunges, look down and make sure your front knee in aligned with your ankle.

-Work in your pain-free range of motion. If your knees don't bend much, don't force it!

SPINAL EXTENSIONS:

1. Lay on your stomach with your hands stacked under your forehead and legs fully extended, reaching toward the wall behind you.
2. With hand remaining in contact with forehead and eye contact remaining on the floor below, slowly lift upper body from the floor to a challenging yet comfortable position. Lift chest up from the floor. If you aren't at that point yet, keep trying to reach this goal.
3. Return upper body to starting position. Repeat 10-15 times.
4. Slowly lift your straight legs from the floor. Make sure this motion is coming from the low back and the glute muscle (the rear end) and NOT the knees. You want to make sure the legs stay straight and reaching toward the wall behind you. Attempt to get some air under the thighs.
5. Return lower body to starting position. Repeat 10-15 times.
6. Lift the upper and lower body at the same time. Repeat 10-15 times.
   Modification: Alternate between upper and lower body.

   Repeat series 2-3 times.

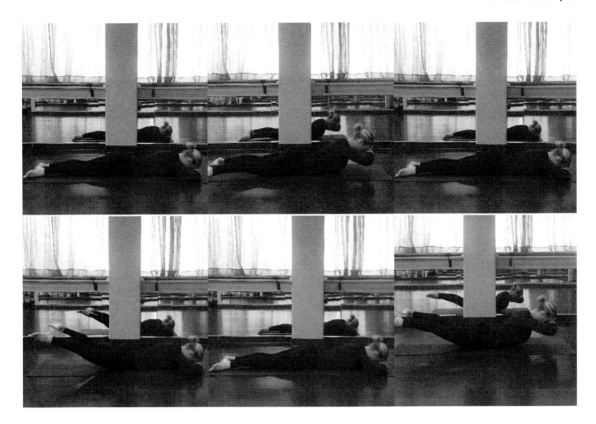

Spinal extension notes:

-*Make sure there is no movement from the neck. All movement should come from the low back and glutes.*

-*Continuously reach your legs long throughout the series. Toes should be pointed; calves, thighs, and glutes should be engaged.*

-*Engage abdominals to stay light in the hip bones. Pressing them into the floor can cause discomfort and takes effort away from the back extensors.*

BRIDGES:

1. Lay on your back and place your feet flat on the floor with your ankles under your knees. Legs will need to be a little wider than your body. Place your arms by your side.
    Modification: If your knees don't allow for that range of motion, bring your feet forward away from the body until you find a comfortable position.

Progression: Lift the heels off of the floor and press the balls of your feet down. Lift arms towards ceiling.

2. Roll the hips up towards the ribcage until the spine is flat on the floor.
3. Engage your glute muscles and lift the hips towards the ceiling.
4. Take 2 counts to relax the glutes and return to starting position by rolling down the spine one vertebra at a time.
5. Take 2 counts to engage the glutes and roll through the spine to return the hips up. Repeat 4-8 times.
6. Continue the same motion, taking 1 count to lower and 1 count to lift the hips. Repeat 8-12 times. Hold at the top of your last lift.
7. Tighten the glutes slightly harder to lift the hips about an inch. Then slightly release the contraction to lower them about an inch. Continue the small pulses 10-14 times.

Repeat series 2-3 times.

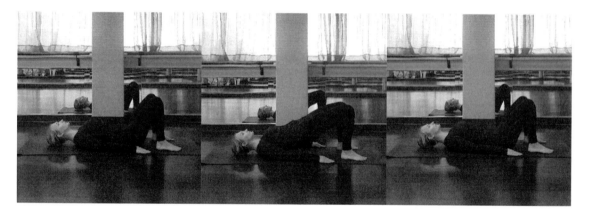

Bridge Notes:

-Create opposition by pressing feet firmly into the floor. This will engage the back of the thighs (your hamstrings).

-You should never feel pressure in your neck. If you do, lower the seat down until you only feel the weight in your upper back.

- Keep your glutes engaged while at the top of your bridge to maximize the benefits of this exercise; only relax the muscles when you return to the floor.

LEG LIFTS:

1. Still lying on your back, bring your legs one at a time to table top position.
2. Roll the hips up towards the ribcage until the spine is fully on the floor.
3. Engage the abdominals to the point of pressing the spine deeply into the floor.
4. Extend your legs to the ceiling and lower the legs forward. Your spine should still be pressed firmly down by the abdominals.
   Modification: Bend at the knees to shorten the lever. If you need support for your low back, place your hands under your tailbone. For more stability, cross at the ankles.
   Progression: Turn out from the hips and press your heels together until you feel your inner thighs engage.
5. Taking four counts, slowly lift your legs back over the hips.
6. Again, for four counts, lower the legs forward stopping before the low back lifts off of the floor. Repeat 5-10 times, holding with your legs lifted after the last repetition.
7. Lower the legs in two counts.
8. Taking two counts, lift the legs to return over the hips. Repeat 5-10 times, holding your legs in the lifted position at the end.
9. Speed up the motion to one count down, and one count up. <u>Please shorten your range of motion to protect your hip joints and back</u>. Repeat 10-15 times.

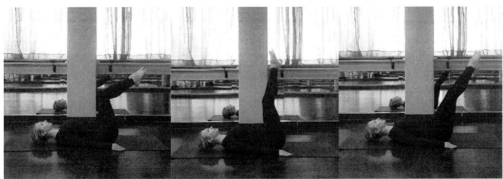

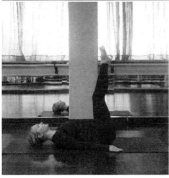

Leg Lift Notes:

-*Make sure you don't hold your breath. Continue breathing! Inhale as you lower the legs, and exhale as you lift them.*

-*If you start to feel your hips gripping or getting tight, bend your knees and shorten your range of motion.*

-*Don't press your arms down into the floor. Make that your abs' job.*

-*Your spine naturally curves, so you'll need to keep your abdominals engaged to keep your spine straight… Stay focused. If you feel your spine starting to come off of the floor, don't lower your legs so far down.*

Congratulations - you've completed your first day of this new program!
Please turn to Page xix for the cool down.

Week One – Day Two

1 Corinthians 6:19-20

> *"Do you not know that your bodies are temples of the Holy Spirit, who is in you, whom you have received from God? You are not your own; you were bought at a price. Therefore, honor God with your bodies."*

Yesterday we read about how our bodies should be considered sacred before the Lord. We know from yesterday's passage that our sacred bodies are temples of the Holy Spirit that moved in when we turned away from sin and turned to Jesus for salvation. Think about an actual temple in biblical times. What took place there? Ritualistic sacrifices at the temple's altar were burned as a form of worship and repentance. We are called to do the same with our flesh. Not burn it, thank goodness, but sacrifice our flesh's desires when they're not in accordance with God's will.

What in your daily life are you willing to sacrifice? What bad habit are you ready to cast away for the glory of God? We don't necessarily need to rid our lives of something for it to be a sacrifice. Think of something you've been postponing; a new healthy habit that you can add to your life. Maybe there is a new form of exercise you've been putting off or something healthy you know you should add to your eating plan. When we put our wishes second to God's, amazing things will happen. God wants us to take care of our bodies, sacrificing certain foods and sloth if need be.

Think about a time when you've been responsible for someone else's belonging; maybe taking care of someone's home, pet, or even a child. We have a tendency to go out of our way and take extra care when we know a loved one is entrusting us with something. In 1 Corinthians, we are reminded that we were bought with a price and we aren't our own. We should take the same special care of these vessels that don't belong to us.

Before we move on to the exercise portion for today, please take a moment to re-read the Bible verse above. As you move about the exercises, allow your mind to focus on the passage. Are there things in your life God is calling you to cast away? Trust in Him and know you can do it. Is there something you want to add to your daily schedule? Make it a priority and trust that God will allow you to find the time, energy, or whatever it is that is holding you back.

DAY TWO FITNESS ROUTINE

Please refer to the warm up on Page xv to prepare your body for today's exercise routine.

CALF RAISES:

1. If needed, stand close to something that can help you balance, a chair for example. With your heels together and toes apart, stretch the spine upwards and engage your abdominals in a baring down motion.
2. Lift the heels off of the floor engaging your calf muscles. Feel the weight dispersed evenly amongst the balls of your feet and all ten toes.
3. Slowly, with control, lower the heels to the floor. Resist the temptation to rock back to your heels. Repeat 8 times.
4. Lift your heels and then only lower half-way down to the floor. Repeat 8 times.
5. Lift your heels and pulse just an inch or so in a bouncing motion. Continue for a count of 16.

Repeat series 2-3 times.

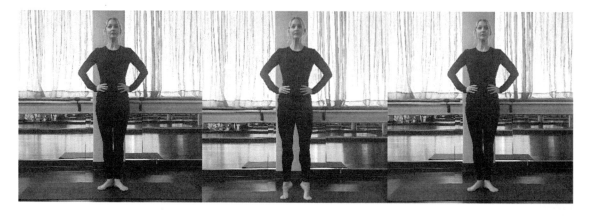

Calf Raise Notes:

-Feel free to take a break when needed and roll the ankle. This exercise will strengthen both the muscle and joint. Honor your body when it needs a break!

-This can also be done in a parallel position with the toes in front of the heels.

*PUSH-UPS:

1. On the floor, place your hands a little wider than your shoulders. Bring your knees back past your hips, not under them. Engage abdominals to support the spine.
   Progression: Attempt push-ups with your knees lifted off of the floor.
   Modification: Push-ups can be done at an angle on a bathroom or kitchen countertop.
2. Slowly bend the elbow to lower the chest towards the floor. Take 3 counts to lower and then lift in 1 count to return to starting position. Three counts down, 1 count up. Repeat 5-10 times.
3. Repeat the movement taking single counts down and up. Repeat as many times as you are able while keeping proper form. *Keep track of the number of repetitions you complete for your "Mile Marker."

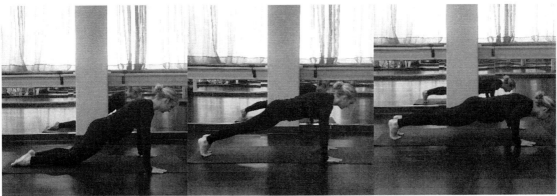

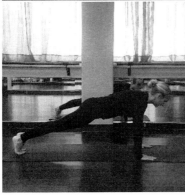

Push-up Notes:

-Be cautious not to drop your head towards the floor. Remember, your head is an extension of the neck which is an extension of the spine.

-Move in your pain-free range of motion. Whatever your joints allow you to accomplish.

-Pictures are in the progression form.

REVERSE CRUNCHES:

1. Lay on your back with your legs lifted towards the ceiling and keep your knees soft. Cross your legs at the ankles and place your hands under your tailbone.
2. Lift your tailbone from the floor and allow it to quickly return down. Do not swing the legs back and forth. It is a quick up and down motion. Repeat 10-15 times.
3. Repeat the movement at a slower pace- 1 count to lift the hips up and 1 count to lower them to the floor. Repeat 5-10 times.

   Repeat series 2-4 times.

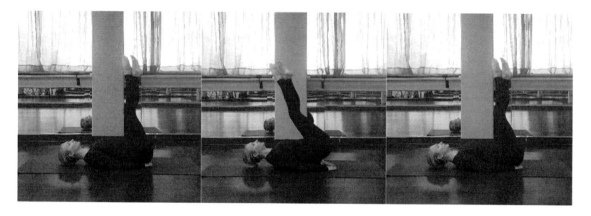

Reverse Crunch Notes:

-Stay light in the arms. Do not press down too hard into the floor. This may cause tension in the neck and shoulders.

-Don't worry about controlling the hips down on the first set. Allow the hips to drop down quickly. The control comes into play when you slow it down on the second round. Feel the spine peel up off of the floor as you lift the hips. Then you use your lower abdominals to control the hips down, lowering one vertebra at a time.

-Watch the angles of your hip and knee joints. Make sure they aren't expanding as you lift your hips. If they are, that simply means you are trying to use momentum from your legs to assist the lift. Allow all the effort to come from your abdominals.

-If your hips start to feel tight, bend your knees more to shorten the lever.

*PLANKS:

1. Start on your knees with either your hands or elbows directly under your shoulders. Bring your knees back past your hips and flex your toes. *Progression: Lift the knees off of the floor.*
2. Engage your abdominals, visualizing hugging your spine so you feel it in your back, sides, and front.
3. Hold the plank position for 60 seconds. *This length of time is at your discretion. If you can't hold it that long yet, do what you can. You WILL eventually get there. If you can go longer than 60 seconds, hold the plank for as long as your body keeps proper form.

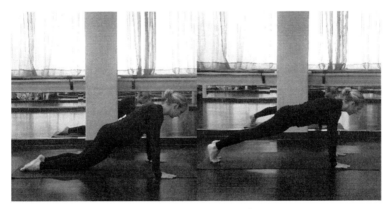

Progression Form

Plank Notes:

-Do not drop your head! Picture a fire under your face… you don't want to get burned!

-Make sure your body is in a nice diagonal line - no mountains with the hips lifted. No valleys with the hips dipped towards the floor.

-Create opposition with the floor. Bare down with either your hands or elbows.

-Last, but most important- KEEP YOUR ABDOMINALS TIGHTLY ENGAGED!

You did it! Great work! Don't forget to turn to Page xix for your cool down.

Week One – Day Three

Romans 12:1

> *"Therefore, I urge you, brothers and sisters, in view of God's mercy, to offer your bodies as a living sacrifice, holy and pleasing to God – this is your true and proper worship."*

Have you given your heart to Jesus Christ? Then why not your whole body? We belong to the Lord – every part of us - mind, heart, soul and body. God does not value our bodies for what they look like, but rather for what they can do. With our bodies, we will complete the assigned tasks we have here on earth. In Romans 6:13 we see again how we are instructed to present ourselves as "instruments of righteousness." Are you able to say, without hesitation, that your body is currently an instrument of righteousness? That it is fully pleasing to God? I know I would personally stumble around my answer to this gut-wrenching question. A physical vessel that is struggling due to lethargy, obesity, or whatever the ailment may be, will have a harder time fulfilling God's callings. Our "yes" may be on the altar, and our hearts are willing, but our bodies may be too weak for the assignment.

Why present our bodies to God as a living sacrifice? Besides the Bible calling us to do so, it is because of what the Lord has done through His grace, mercy, and love. We are free because of His example of being a literal living sacrifice. Jesus offered himself up as the unblemished lamb, the ultimate sacrifice, so we may spend forever with Him. So really, the question should be – WHY NOT? I know this sounds like a tall order, but this fitness devotional is designed to help you every step of the way.

Remove the pressure of having to be a perfect, self-sacrificing individual; that is not what this is about. I'm not suggesting that you completely void your life of all pleasure. Simply take time to think about what you put into your body and what you do with your it. Is it beneficial for your health? Will it help you live a life fulfilling God's calling? If not, change your course of action and do so for the glory of God. Don't be intimidated, be inspired. This is the beginning of your new journey and it's bigger than you, bigger than any fitness goals you've ever imagined, and I am so excited to see how the Lord will work in your heart during the next month.

Before we move on to the exercise portion for today, please take a moment to re-read the Bible verse above. As you move about the exercises, allow your mind to focus on the passage and on what it means for you at this point in your life. In what ways can you honor God with your body?

DAY THREE FITNESS ROUTINE – HAND WEIGHTS

Start with heavier weights and feel free to move to a lighter weight at any point. Weights are not required but recommended to maximize your results.

Please refer to the warmup on Page 6 to prepare your body for today's exercise routine.

WEIGHTED FLIES:

1. Stand with your feet hip distance apart, bend knees, and hinge forward from the hips. Engage abdominals to support your spine. Depress shoulders down the back. Allow your eyes to focus on the floor a few feet in front of you to keep the neck long. With your weights in hand, hug an imaginary beach ball in front of your chest.
2. Take 2 counts to open the arms to the sides as if the beach ball is getting bigger. Feel the shoulder blades moving towards the spine.
3. Take 2 counts to lower the arms to starting position. Repeat 8 times.
4. Repeat the same movement taking single counts to lift and lower the arms. Repeat 8 times.
5. Lift arms to your highest comfortable position and pulse the arms half-way down. Repeat 16 times.

Repeat series 1-3 times.

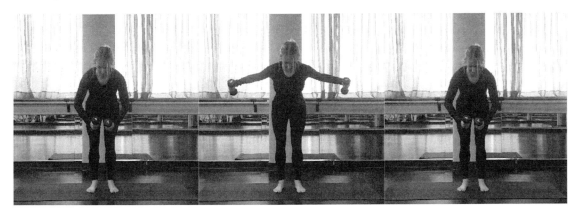

Weighted Fly Notes:

-*Be cautious not to allow the abdominals to disengage. This will cause the spine to drop and create tension in the low back.*

-*While lowering the shoulder blades down the spine, reach the ears away from the shoulders to keep the neck long.*

-*Move in your pain-free range of motion.*

-*Keep the body's weight in your heels. You should be able to wiggle your toes.*

SIDE BICEP CURLS:

1. Stand with your feet hip distance apart and core engaged. Bring your elbows to your ribcage with your palms facing up.
2. Extend your arms to the sides and lift your elbows to shoulder height. *Modification: Lift your elbows only as high as comfortable if you have shoulder discomfort.*
3. Flex at the elbow joint, bringing the hands towards the shoulders.
4. Extend the arms back out.
5. Lower the elbows back to the ribcage. Repeat 10-15 times.
6. Shortening your range of motion (not lifting as high), pulse the extension of the arms; quickly extending the arms and then quickly returning them to the ribcage. Repeat 10-15 times.

Repeat series 2-4 times.

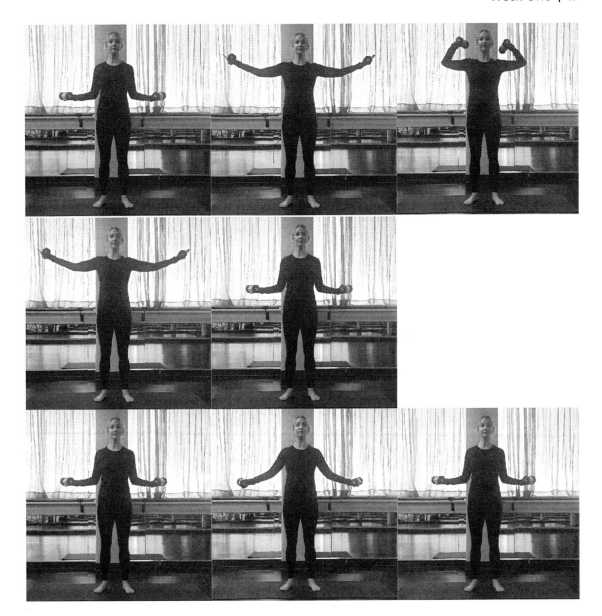

Side Bicep Curl Notes:

-When you lift and extend the arms, keep your abdominals tight and your ribcage pulled in towards the spine.

-Work in your pain-free range of motion.

-Stay strong in the wrists. Don't allow the weight to pull the knuckles down.

TRICEP SERIES:

1. Stand with your feet hip distance apart, bend knees, hinge forward from the hips. Engage abdominals to support spine. Depress shoulders down the back. Allow your eyes to focus on the floor a few feet in front of you to keep the neck long. Extend your arms under the shoulders, palms facing each other.
2. Lift your arms behind, hold, and reach them long behind you to properly engage the back of the arm. *Modification: Lower the arms behind to ease shoulder discomfort.*
3. Lower the arms to return to starting position. Repeat 10-15 times.
4. Lift the arms behind, palms facing in, and without lowering the elbow, bend your arms to bring the hand towards the shoulders.
5. Extend back to starting position. Repeat 10-15 times.

Repeat series 2-3 times.

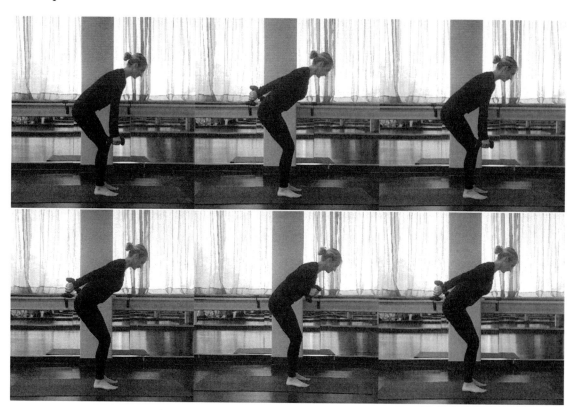

Tricep Series Notes:

- Keep the abs tight and the spine straight. Don't allow it to dip towards to the floor as this will cause lower back tension.

- Work in your pain-free range of motion.

-To fully maximize the benefits of these exercises, fully extend and reach the arms long behind you.

-Your body weight should be in your heels, allowing you to wiggle your toes freely.

WEIGHTED EXTENSIONS:

1. Lay on your back, weights in hands. Extend the arms to the ceiling right above the shoulders with palms facing in. Bring both legs to a table top position. Imprint your spine on the floor; roll the hips up towards the ribcage and contract the abdominals to firmly press the spine into the floor.
2. Take 2 counts to extend the right leg in front and lower the left arm towards the head. Keep the limb off of the floor. Do not allow the spine to come up from the floor.
    Modification: For shoulder discomfort, limit the range of motion in the arms. You may also bend at the knees and elbows to shorten the length of your limbs.
3. Take 2 counts to bring leg and arm back to starting position.
4. Repeat on opposite side.

    Repeat on each side 8-15 times.

    Progression: Continue the same movement but speeding it up to 1 count for each movement
    Rest if needed and repeat series 2-3 times.

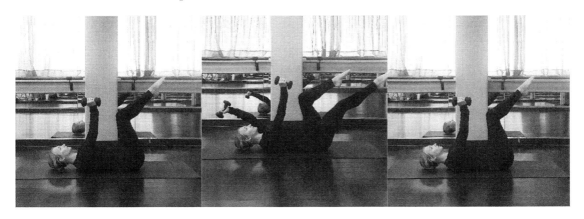

Weighted Extensions Notes:

- If you feel your abdominals releasing and the spine leaving the floor, lift your leg higher when you extend it.

-Move in your pain-free range of motion.

-If hips start to feel tight, don't fully extend the legs.

Great job! You've completed Day Three! Turn to Page xix for your cool down.

Week One – Day Four

Philippians 1:20

> *"I eagerly expect and hope that I will in no way be ashamed, but will have sufficient courage so that now as always Christ will be exalted in my body, whether by life or by death."*

Like Paul, we too should strive to courageously exalt Christ with our bodies. Our hopes and expectations can now escape the demands of our modern culture. Social media, advertisements, and even some cartoons have shaped the way we look at our bodies and what we expect them to be able to achieve. It is exhausting trying to keep up with an unrealistic idealization. Take rest in the knowledge that our bodies need to do only one thing- exalt our Heavenly Father.

The good news is that we don't need six-pack abdominals or have to bench press three hundred pounds to do so. We simply need to take care of our earthly vessels so we may pursue what God calls us to do. We will all have different assignments. Mine has taken me on a whirlwind of a ride becoming a fitness instructor and author – two things I never had planned for myself.

I love that Paul mentioned not being ashamed and having courage. He didn't just mention it; he hoped for and expected it. It leads me to believe that Paul prayed many times for this. I have been in his shoes and I bet many of you have as well; praying for strength and courage.

Before I was in the fitness industry, I was in finance. I was a loan officer at a local bank and I worked hard to hold that position. In the time before tendering my resignation to become a stay-at-home mom, I felt like I was constantly praying for the strength it would take to leave all that I had worked so hard to achieve. I didn't feel ashamed of my decision. I did however feel like I was letting a part of myself down, but I knew that wasn't where God was calling me. I prayed for strength and courage to follow His path and not my own. I can honestly tell you that I have never looked back.

It takes a lot of strength and courage to make any change in your life. For some of you, this program is a massive alteration. Having quiet time with the Lord, reading a devotional, and exercising six days a week! And for some of you, this may be a nice addition to an already full personal regime. Either way, it took being unashamed of wanting to improve yourself and your relationship with God to open this book. Good job!

Before we move on to the exercise portion for today, please take a moment to re-read the Bible verse above. As you move about the exercises, allow your mind to focus on the passage. Have there been times in your life when it took being unashamed and courageous to exalt God? Are you currently weary or nervous about something? Give it to the Lord and be ready to be amazed at what He will do with it.

DAY FOUR FITNESS ROUTINE

Please refer to the warm up on Page xv to prepare your body for today's exercise routine.

*BICYCLE OBLIQUE CRUNCHES:

1. Lay on your back and bring both legs to table top position. Spread out your fingertips, cradle the back of your head, and bring the elbows away from the face. Lift your head and shoulder blades from the floor. Imprint your spine onto the floor.
2. Extend your right leg to the ceiling and lower it to a comfortable level where the spine is still in contact with the floor. *Modification: Keep both legs bent with feet flat on the floor.*
3. Rotate the upper body bringing the right shoulder towards the left knee. Hold for a count of 4.
4. Switch sides. Return the right leg to table top and extend the left leg in front. Rotate the upper body bringing the left shoulder towards the right knee. Hold for a count of 4. Repeat at this pace 4-8 times on each side.
5. Continue the same movement holding the crunch for 2 counts on each side. Repeat 6-10 times on each side.
6. Continue the bicycle motion speeding up the crunch hold for 1 count on each side. Repeat 8-12 times on each side.

   *Progression: *Move through the bicycle motion as fast as you can while keeping good form. Continue the "cardio cycle" for as long as you can. Keep track of your time and use this progression as a "Mile Marker."*

   Repeat series 1-3 times.

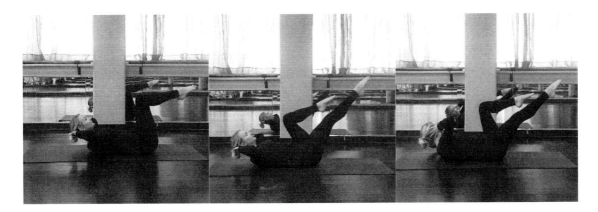

Bicycle Oblique Crunch Notes:

-Allow your elbows to be seen in your peripheral vision. If they are too wide, it can cause straining in the neck and shoulders. If the elbows are too close to the face, you're probably pulling on the neck causing unnecessary tension.

-If your hips start to feel tight, don't fully extend your legs.

-Make sure it's the shoulder and not the elbow that is aiming towards the knee. This will ensure proper oblique engagement.

-Allow the weight of your head to fully rest in your hands to minimize neck discomfort.

WIDE LEG BRIDGES:

1. Lay on your back and place your feet flat on the floor with your ankles under your knees. Open your legs as wide as your comfortly can. Turn out from the hips. Your toes should be facing diagonal. Place your arms by your side.
   Modification: If your knees don't allow for that range of motion, bring your feet forward until you find a comfortable position.
   Progression: Lift the heels off of the floor and press the balls of your feet down. Lift arms towards ceiling
2. Roll the hips up towards the ribcage until the spine is flat on the floor.
3. Engage your glute muscles and lift the hips towards the ceiling.
4. Using your outer glutes and thighs, take 2 counts to gently pull the knees out wider.
5. Using your inner thighs, control the motion as you take 2 counts to come back into the starting position. Repeat at this pace 8-10 times.

6. Continue the same out-and-in motion but speed it up to 1 count out and 1 count in. Repeat at this pace 15-20 times.
7. With the same movement, work in a smaller range of motion to pulse the knees out and in. Repeat pulses 15-20 times.

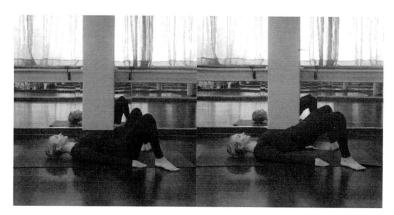

Wide Bridge Notes:

-If your low back needs support, place a pillow under the back or set the seat back on the floor. The motions are still effective in this position as well.

LEG LIFT SCISSORS:

1. Laying on your back, bring your legs one at a time to table top position.
2. Imprint the spine; roll the hips up towards the ribcage until the spine is fully on the floor. Engage the abdominals to the point of pressing the spine deeply into the floor.
3. Extend your legs to the ceiling and lower the legs forward. Your spine should still be pressed firmly down by the abdominals. (This is your full range of motion.) *Modification: Bend at the knees to shorten the lever. If you need support for your low back, place your hands under your tailbone. Progression: Reach your arms towards the ceiling.*
4. Return the legs back to the ceiling.
5. Take 4 counts to lower the right leg towards the floor. If your spine begins to come off of the floor, you've lowered too far.
6. Take 4 counts to return the leg over the hip.
7. Repeat on left side. Repeat at this pace 2-4 times on each side.
8. Take 2 counts to lower the right leg towards the floor.
9. Take 2 counts to return the leg towards the ceiling.
10. Repeat on left side. Repeat at this pace 2-4 times on each side.

11. Shortening your range of motion, take 1 count to lower the right leg towards the floor.
12. Take 1 count to return the leg over the hip.
13. Repeat on left side. Repeat at this pace 2-4 times on each side.

    Repeat series 2-3 times.

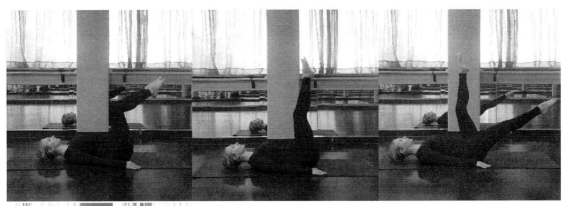

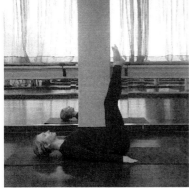

Leg Lift Scissor Notes:
-It is extremely easy to want to hold your breath during this exercise. Remember to breathe in through the nose and out through the mouth.

*TRICEP PUSH-UPS:

1. Starting on all fours, place your hands directly under the shoulders with the fingers pointing forward. Bring your knees back past your hips. Engage the core so the spine does not dip towards the floor. Your neck is long.
   Progression: Lift the knees from the floor into a full push-up position.

2. Taking 3 counts, bend at the elbows allowing the arms to brush the sides of your body as your torso lowers towards the floor.
3. Take a single count to extend the arms to return to starting position. Repeat 4-6 times.
4. Reverse the counts. Take 1 count to lower the body and 3 counts to extend at the elbow to raise the body. Repeat 4-6 times.
5. Continue the same motion, taking 1 count down and 1 count to come up. Repeat as many times as you can while keeping proper form.

Repeat series 1-3 times.

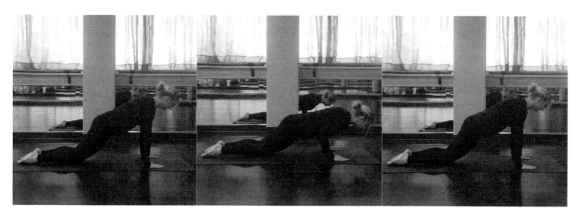

Tricep Push-up Notes:

-*Due to the difficulty level of this exercise, the number of repetitions you are able to complete is your "Mile Marker."

-Do not drop your head towards the floor.

-Keep the abdominals engaged to support the spine.

-Tell yourself to squeeze your ribs with your elbows. This will help you keep the arms close to the body.

-Allow the elbows to bend in such a way that they are "pointing" in the direction of your toes.

Your body is getting stronger. Congratulations! Remember your cool down on Page xix.

Week One – Day Five

1 Samuel 16:7

> *"But the Lord said to Samuel, 'Do not consider his appearance or his height, for I have rejected him. The Lord does not look at the things people look at. People look at the outward appearance, but the Lord looks at the heart'."*

It is what's on the inside that counts! We have heard that a thousand times growing up. It was a good lesson then and it is a good lesson now. What is in your heart? What fuels you? If your motives aren't pure in this program or in general, you won't maximize your results in anything you put your efforts into.

Push vanity and selfish ambitions aside. This isn't about looking a certain way, seeing a certain number on the scale, or being able to do a certain amount of repetitions at the gym. This BOW program is about devoting your body to the Lord. (Isn't that acronym a beautiful illustration? BOW- humbling ourselves before the Lord). It is also about learning and honoring our bodies so we are capable of completing the tasks God puts in front of us.

When God looks at you, He doesn't notice your outward appearance. He doesn't care about the length of your hair, how fit you are, or what you are wearing. He looks to the beauty of your heart. Honestly, how relieving is that? The one and only judge does not care what you look like! I can almost hear the drawers slamming shut as you grab for your sweat pants right now. No, we don't exercise and eat well to impress the Lord, or anyone for that matter. We do so in order to properly execute what the Lord calls us to do.

Now let's flip this around – what do you look at in yourself and in others? Yikes, another gut-wrenching question! Are you like me and are easier on others than you are on yourself? You are your own worst critic- another classic saying. Bestow some of that grace you share with others onto yourself. We will dive deeper into this topic later in Chapter Three. For now, focus on what you've already learned: your body is sacred, it is a temple for the Holy Spirit, and it is a living sacrifice to the Lord. That is just a quick snapshot of what the Lord sees when He looks at you and I pray you start to see yourself in that light as well.

Before we move on to the exercise portion for today, please take a moment to re-read the Bible verse above. As you move about the exercises, allow your mind to focus on the qualities you admire about yourself- nothing physical but the qualities of your heart.

DAY FIVE FITNESS ROUTINE

Please refer to the warm up on Page xv to prepare your body for today's exercise routine.

*BURPEES:

1. Stand with your legs wider than your body.
2. Bend the knees, and bring your hands to the floor directly under the shoulders.
3. Step back with the right leg to bring it directly behind the right hip. Repeat with the left leg. You will end up in a plank formation.
   Progression: Hop both legs out simultaneously into plank position and add a push up.
4. Step right leg up and then back to its starting position. Repeat with the left leg to end in a tuck position. *Progression: Hop both legs back in at the same time.*
5. Stand up.

Repeat as many times as you can without losing proper form.

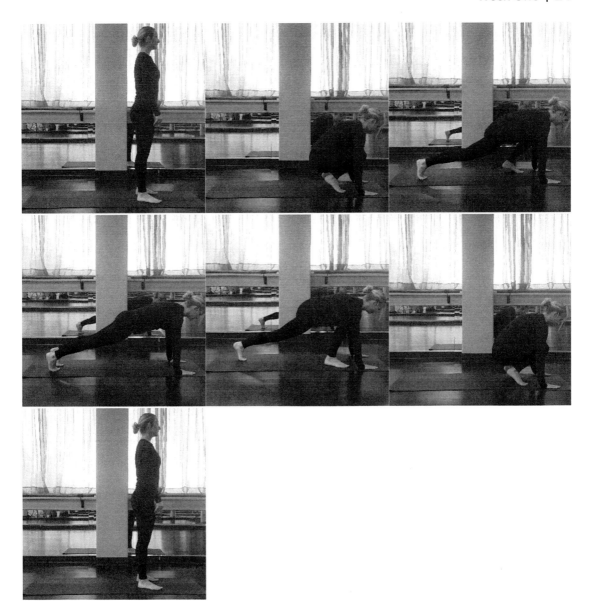

Burpee Notes:

-This can be a higher intensity exercise. If your body does not like this move for whatever reason, please replace this exercise with a previous one from earlier in the week.

-Keep track of the number of repetitions you complete. The number of reps completed will be your "Mile Marker."

-Go at your comfortable pace. Remember, you want to push yourself-not hurt yourself!

PLIÉ SQUATS:

1. Stand with your legs wider than your body, hips turned out and toes pointing diagonally. Engage the core, proud chest with shoulders low down the spine. Reach the top of your head towards the ceiling.
   Modification: Feel free to use a chair or another prop to help you with your balance if needed.
   Progression: Lift the heels from the floor and balance on the balls of your feet.
2. Neutralize the hips by rolling them up towards the ribcage. The tailbone should point towards the floor, not behind you.
3. Take 4 counts to bend the knees to your lowest comfortable position. Feel the outer glutes and thighs engage as the knees pull outward slightly to track over the toes.
4. Take 4 counts to extend the legs back to starting position. Repeat 8-10 times.
5. Take 2 counts to lower into your plie position.
6. Take 2 counts to extend the legs. Repeat 8-10 times.
7. Hold at your lowest comfortable position and quickly pulse a slight extension, lifting just a couple of inches, and lower back down. Repeat 15-20 times.

Repeat series 2-4 times.

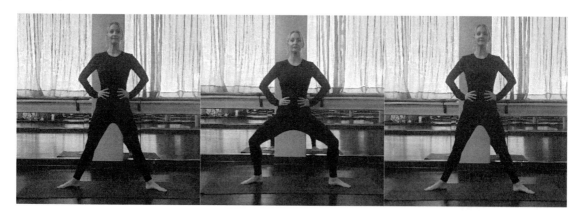

Plié Squat Notes:

-Imagine your upper back moving down and up an imaginary wall behind you. You want to keep your head over the shoulders and shoulders over the hips.

-Be aware of hinging forward. This is common but not proper form. Hinging and loosening of the abdominals often causes the hips to tilt forward. Keep the pelvic region neutral. You'll feel the natural curve in your low back minimize when done correctly.

-Watch your knees. Make sure they are tracking over the toes.

SIDE PLANK:

1. Lay on your right side with your elbow on the floor under the shoulder. Palm on the floor. Left hand on your left hip. Bend your bottom leg to a comfortable position. Top leg extended straight.
   Progression: Place your hand under your shoulder with your right arm straight. For further intensity, you may also keep both legs extended with top foot staggered on the floor in front of bottom foot.
2. Using your abdominals, take 2 counts to lift your hips from the floor. Extend your left arm up and reach overhead. Look up towards your fingers.
3. Lower the hips back towards the floor in 2 counts. Hand returns to hip. Repeat 8-10 times.
4. Repeat on the other side. Repeat 8-10 times.

   Repeat series 2-3 times.

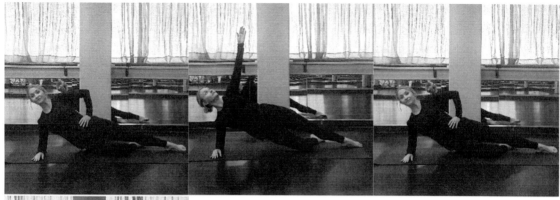

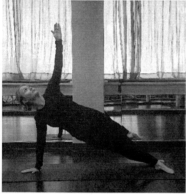

Progression Form

Side Plank Notes:

-Don't allow the head to drop towards the shoulder. You want to keep your neck extended to prevent tension.

-Engage the bottom oblique abdominals to properly lift the hips and ribcage.

SPINAL EXTENSION SUPERMAN:

1. Lay on your stomach with your arms extended straight in front. Extend the legs behind.
   Modification: Bend your arms at the elbows to relieve any shoulder tension. For further ease, allow the arms to remain on the floor.
2. Take 2 counts to lift the arms and upper body from the floor. Keep movement out of the neck. Make sure all lifting is coming from the low back and glutes.
3. Take 2 counts to return to starting position.
4. Take 2 counts to lift the legs from the floor.
5. Take 2 counts to lower the legs to starting position.

6. Repeat 4-6 times.
7. Take a single count to lift the arms and chest from the floor.
8. Take a single count to lower back down.
9. Repeat with the lower body.
10. Repeat 4-6 times.
11. Lift the upper body then the lower body. Hold both at the top for 15-30 seconds.
12. Lower back to the floor and rock the hips side to side to relax the lower back.

Repeat series 2-3 times.

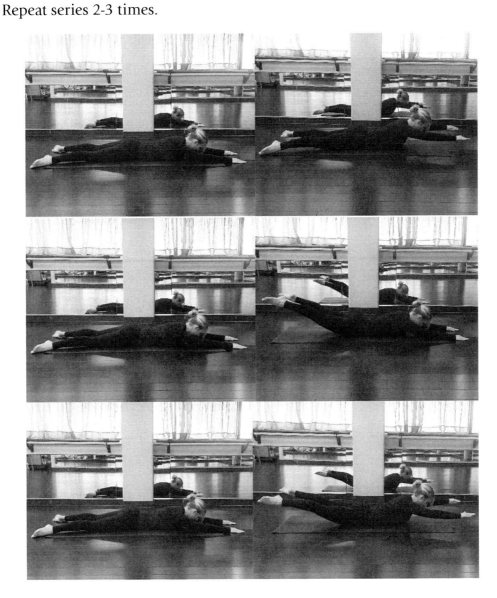

Spinal Extension Superman Notes:

-Focus on the extension of the legs. Allow them to reach and stretch behind you. You should feel the entire leg engage.

-Keep the shoulders from tensing up and moving up towards the ears. Press them low down the spine.

Are you feeling stronger yet? Go to Page xix to reference your cool down if needed.

Week One – Day Six

1 Timothy 4:8

> *"For physical training is of some value, but godliness has value for all things, holding promise for both the present life and the life to come."*

Some might read this verse and at first glance, celebrate that the Bible says exercise isn't that important. But as you dig deeper, it speaks a different message. Yes, physical training has value here on earth. If we look towards heavenly rewards, that value diminishes.

Does having the ability to run a 10K race get you closer to Heaven's gate? Of course not! By all means, train for that race if that is important to you, but find the strength and endurance the run requires in the Lord. Finish your goal knowing God was there fueling you. Do you have a goal you're working towards? Share it with God and allow Him to help you. When you succeed, to God be the glory! Having earthly goals is not a bad thing, but it shouldn't be everything. Keep your eyes on the ultimate goal – eternal life in Heaven.

During the time Paul was writing to Timothy, the ancient greek and Roman culture placed much significance on athletic training; similar to our culture today. But what Paul was emphasizing to Timothy was that the amount of effort athletes put into their training, they should also put into their pursuit of godliness. How much effort and energy do you put into your earthly goals? Is it matched by the amount you put into your heavenly goals?

Before we move on to the exercise portion for today, please take a moment to re-read the Bible verse above. As you move about the exercises, allow your mind to focus on some heavenly goals you can work towards. Some options may be improving your prayer life, showing gratitude, or spreading the gospel. As you focus on a goal, think about how you can put mental and physical energy into your training that would parallel an athlete's efforts.

DAY SIX FITNESS ROUTINE

Please refer to the warm up on Page xv to prepare your body for today's exercise routine.

BIRD-DOG SERIES:

1. Begin on all fours; hands under shoulders and knees under hips. Abdominals engaged and spine straight. Keep your neck long, don't allow the head to drop towards the floor.
2. Extend your right leg on the floor behind you and slowly lift the leg to your highest point where the back does not begin to dip towards the floor.
3. Once you feel balanced, slowly lift the opposite arm, the left arm, to shoulder height.
4. Extend the arm long in front and the leg long behind. Balance here for 20-30 seconds.
   Modification: If needed, feel free to lift only the arm or only the leg.
5. Moving in the hip and shoulder joints, lower the leg and arm simultaneously to tap the floor.
6. Lift limbs to return to starting position. Repeat 8-10 times.
7. Take 2 counts to open the leg to the right, keeping the leg as high as possible.
8. Take 2 counts to open the arm to the left, attempting to remain at shoulder height.
9. Take 2 counts to return the leg behind the hip.
10. Take 2 counts to return the arm in front of the shoulder.
    Progression: Move both the arm and the leg to the sides at the same time. Repeat 4-6 times.
11. Repeat series on the opposite side; left leg and right arm.

    Repeat series on both sides 2-3 times.

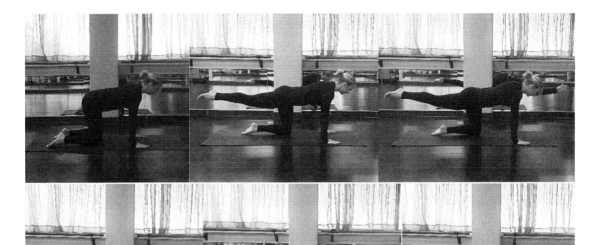

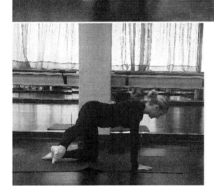

Bird-Dog Notes:

-Core engagement is vital for stabilization. Keep the ribcage and bellybutton pulled in to the spine. Remember, it is not a "suck in" motion but rather a "bearing down" motion.

-Make sure the spine does not dip towards the floor. If you notice you're having a hard time with this, don't lift the limbs as high.

-Notice how the standing arm and legs work hard in the shoulder and hip areas to stabilize. Without even moving, those muscles are strengthening.

-To relieve any wrist tension, lower your elbows onto the floor.

-Be mindful that the movements continue to come from the hip and shoulder joints. As your body becomes tired, it may want to move in the elbows and knees. This will not maximize your efforts.

TRIANGLE LEG LIFTS:

1. Lay on your right side, your right arm extended under the head. Stack your hips, knees, and ankles. Bring your legs slightly in front of you. Left hand on the floor in front of your chest to help with stability.
   Modification: Bend your bottom leg to increase support and stability.
2. Engage your core. You should feel it in your front, sides, and back.
3. Lengthen your top leg and lift it towards the ceiling.
4. Keeping the hips stacked, take 2 counts to lower the leg diagonally to the floor in front of you.
5. Take 2 counts to return the leg up towards the ceiling and back in line with your body.
6. Keeping the hips stacked, take 2 counts to lower the leg diagonally to the floor behind you.
   Modification: If you're unable to contact the floor, just go to your lowest comfortable point.
7. Take 2 counts to return the leg to the ceiling and back in line with the body. Repeat 4-6 times.
8. Take a single count to lower the leg diagonally to the floor in front of you.
9. Take a single count to return the leg up towards the ceiling.
10. In a single count, lower the leg diagonally to the floor behind you.
11. Take 1 count to return the leg to the ceiling and back in line with the body. Repeat 10-15 times.
    Modification: With the pace speeding up, you may need to shorten your range of motion to protect your joints. As always, move in your pain-free range of motion.
12. Repeat the series on the left side.

    Repeat series on both sides 1-3 times.

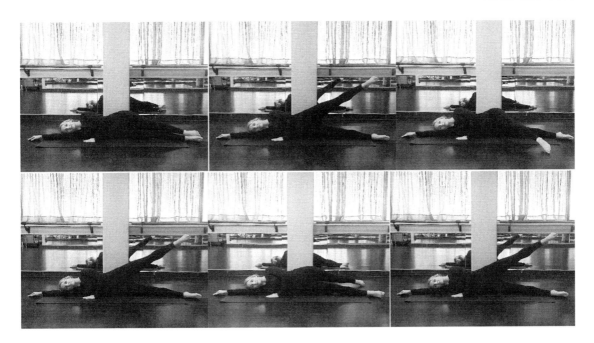

Triangle Leg Lift Notes:

-As the name implies, you are drawing a triangle shape with your leg. I have found it helpful to close my eyes and picture the triangle. Imagine yourself tracing the triangle with your big toe.

-The top arm is there to support you but don't let it be your only form of support. Your abdominals should be doing most of the stabilizing.

-If your bottom leg is straight, make sure you are lengthening it as well as the top leg. You should feel your quadriceps (your top thigh) and your calves engage.

GOLDEN ARCHES:

1. Lay on your stomach with your hands stacked on the floor and your forehead on top of your hands. Allow your hips to naturally turn out, lengthen your legs and bring them close together. Visualize a big "m" behind you. Much like the sign for a popular fast food chain.
2. Using your low back and glutes, lift your legs from the floor.
3. Moving in an arch pattern to trace the "m" behind you, take 2 counts to lift, open, and then tap the toes on the floor.
4. Again taking 2 counts, lift the legs and in the same arch pattern, allow them to come back into their starting position close to each other on the floor.
5. Continue to trace the big "m" at the two-count pace 4-6 times.

6. Now imagine the big "m" gets smaller and use a quicker one-count pace to trace it.
7. Take 1 count to lift up and move out. Take 1 count to lift up and come back in.

Repeat series 2-4 times.

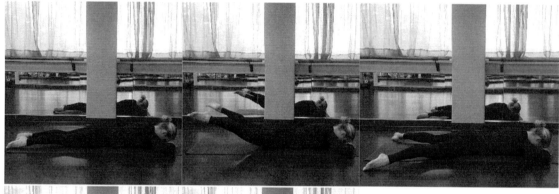

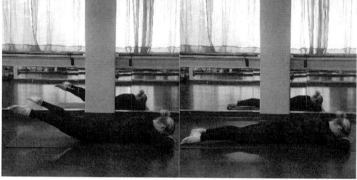

Golden Arches Notes:

-This move does require some coordination; it may take some practice so be patient with yourself. Keep imagining you're tracing the infamous golden arches with your big toe. And yes, I know it is mean of me to make you think of fast food while you're working out. I'm sorry.

-Engage the abdominals to stay light in the hips.

-Keep your head on your stacked hands to have proper spinal alignment.

KNEE DROP PLANKS:

1. Start on the floor with either your hands or elbows directly under your shoulders. Bring your knees back past your hips and flex your toes. Lift your knees off of the floor. *Modification: If you are not able to hold your full plank yet, keep the knees on the floor. You will hold your knee plank instead of continuing with the Knee Drop version.*

2. Engage your abdominals. Visualize hugging your spine so you feel it in your back, sides, and front.
3. Lower the right knee to tap the floor.
4. Lift the knee back in line to full plank position. Repeat on the right side 5-10 times.
5. Lower the left knee to tap the floor.
6. Return the knee to full plank position. Repeat on left side 5-10 times.
7. At the same time, bring both knees to tap the floor.
8. Lift both knees back to plank. Repeat 4-8 times.

Repeat series 2-3 times.

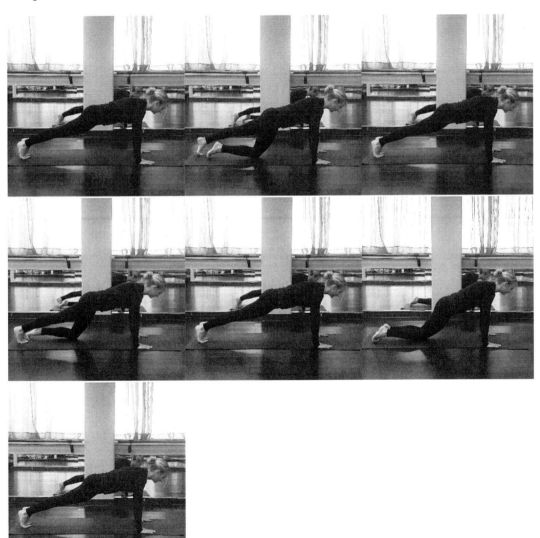

Knee Drop Plank Notes:

-*Do not drop your head towards the floor.*

-*Make sure your body is in a nice diagonal line…. No mountains with the hips lifted. No valleys with the hips dipped towards the floor.*

-*Create opposition with the floor by baring down with either your hands or elbows.*

-*If you need to take a quick break in between rounds, please do.*

-*Finally, but most important- KEEP YOUR ABDOMINALS TIGHTLY ENGAGED!*

You have successfully completed your first week of *A Body of Worship.* Way to Go!

Turn to Page xix for the cool down.

WEEK TWO

A Body of Worship has self-control and self-discipline.

Week Two – Day One

2 Timothy 1:7

> *"For the Spirit God gave us does not make us timid, but gives us power, love, and self-discipline."*

This verse is short and sweet, but the message is strong and empowering. Everything you need to strive was placed inside of you when the Holy Spirit took up residence in your heart.

What are the characteristics that come to mind when you think of a timid person? Shy, weak, maybe even a coward? These are things we are NOT! Yes, of course, some of us may be shy but that doesn't mean we shy away from challenges. We are powerful, loving, and self-disciplined creatures. This is not of our own doing but a spiritual gift from God. When things get hard; when temptations cause us to struggle, we can still have confidence. We can have confidence in the self-discipline and power that was gifted to us by our Creator. As believers, we all have the strength it takes to control our flesh's cravings and urges. How relieving is that? You and I have the capability to stare down our temptations and come out even stronger on the other side.

Before we move on to today's fitness routine, please re-read the Bible verse and let it really sink in. How does that make you feel - knowing that what you need is already in you? Take some time to reflect on what really tempts you in your day-to-day life. The things that used to have power over you are now weakened by the power and self-discipline gifted by God.

DAY ONE FITNESS ROUTINE

Please refer to the warm up on Page xv to prepare your body for today's exercise routine.

*PUSH-UPS:

1. On the floor, place your hands a little wider than your shoulders. Bring your knees past your hips, not under them. Engage abdominals to support the spine. *Attempt push-ups with your knees lifted off of the floor.
   Modification: Push-ups can be done at an angle on a bathroom or kitchen countertop.

2. Slowly bend the elbow to lower the chest towards the floor. Take 3 counts to lower and then lift in 1 count to return to starting position. Three counts down, 1 count up. Repeat 5-10 times.

3. Repeat the movement taking single counts down and up. Repeat as many times as possible while keeping proper form. *Keep track of your number of repetitions for your "Mile Marker."

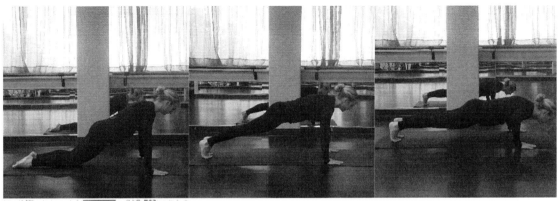

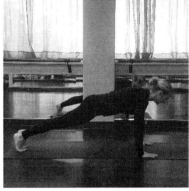

Push-up Notes:

-Don't drop your head towards the floor. Remember, your head is an extension of the neck which is an extension of the spine.

-Move in your pain-free range of motion. Whatever your joints allow you to accomplish.

-Pictures are shown in the progression form.

CAN-CAN:

1. Start by sitting up straight. Lean back to place your elbows on the floor under your shoulders. Palms flat on the floor. Engage the core. Bend your legs and press your knees and ankles together. Lift up your heels and place your big toes on the floor. Bring your toes as close to your seat as your knees will comfortably allow. Toes should be lined up with the middle of your body.
   Progression: Extend the legs to bring the toes further from the body.
2. Moving from the hips, lift your toes from the floor and twist your hips over to the right then lower the right baby toe back down to the same spot.
3. Lift the legs and rotate to the left. Lower the left baby-toe to the same spot in the middle of your body. Repeat 10-15 times on each side.
4. Rest if needed and repeat the series 2-3 times.

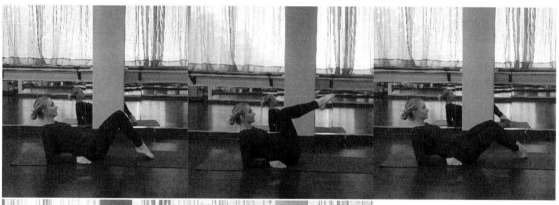

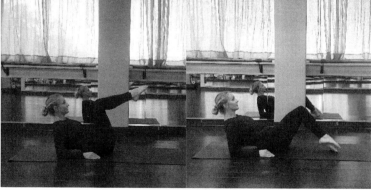

Can-Can Notes:

-*Imagine a penny on the floor in line with the middle of your body. As you lower your baby-toes towards the floor, aim to touch that imaginary penny each time. The penny does not move.*

-*Keep the abdominals engaged to allow the spine to stay in proper alignment. The spine should remain lifted, straight, and not curved forward.*

-*If your hips are feeling tight, keep the toes closer to the body.*

-*Press the forearms into the floor to lift up out of your shoulder girdle. Don't slump into your shoulders.*

-*Keep your chin lifted from your chest so the airway is open.*

-*Keep your knees in contact with one another.*

SUMO-SQUATS:

1. Stand with your feet a little wider than your hips. Hands pressed together in front of the chest in prayer position. Elbows lifted to be in line with wrists.
2. Hinge forward from the hips and bend at the knees to your lowest comfortable level.
3. Lift the upper body and extend the legs to return to standing position.
4. Lift the right leg to the side.
5. Lower the leg to return back to the floor. Repeat 5 times.
6. Repeat the series lifting the left leg. Repeat 5 times.

   Repeat series 2-3 times.

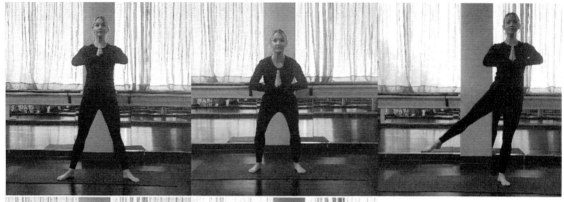

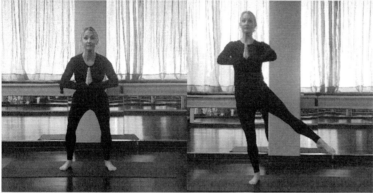

Sumo-Squat Notes:

-While bending the knees, look down and make sure they are tracking over the toes.

-Keep the core engaged to support the spinal movement.

-Press the hands firmly together to engage the upper body.

-While lifting the leg, keep your torso over the hips. Don't allow the body to lean over to the opposite side.

-Lower the leg with control. Allow the inner thigh to control the movement.

STRADDLE LEG LIFTS:

1. Lay on your back with your legs in table-top position, arms on the floor by your sides. Imprint your spine onto the floor by rolling your hips towards your ribcage and compressing the abdominals. There should be no arch in the spine. Extend your legs towards the ceiling.
    Modification: If you need support for your lower back, place hands under tailbone.

2. Take 2 counts to lower the legs outward to a straddle position.
3. Take 2 counts to lift the legs, bringing them back towards each other. Repeat 4-6 times.
4. Take 1 count to lower into straddle.
5. Take 1 count to lift back together. Repeat 6-8 times.

   Repeat series 2-3 times.

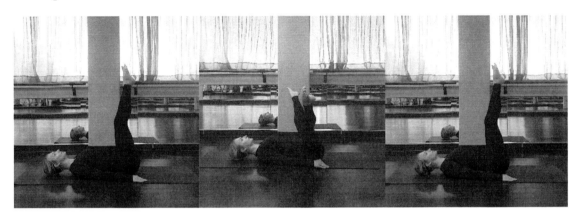

Straddle Leg Lift Notes:

-Keep your knees soft so the fronts of your thighs don't contract.

-Make sure the spine doesn't leave the floor.

-Move in your pain-free range of motion.

-To relieve any tension in the hips, bend slightly more at the knees.

Cool down time and it is well deserved!

Week Two – Day Two

1 Corinthians 10:13

> *"No temptation has overtaken you except what is common to mankind. And God is faithful; he will not let you be tempted beyond what you can bear. But when you are tempted, he will also provide a way out so that you can endure it."*

Don't you feel like you can take a big sigh of relief after reading that? I know I do! The Bible doesn't say life will be easy as Christians. In fact, it is quite the opposite. The enemy is constantly lurking around the corner just waiting to attack with all sorts of temptations and trickery. He is watching and knows about your new adventure with *A Body of Worship.* So be prepared for his lies and deceit. I can hear the whispers now, "Is it really dishonoring God if you take a day off from your devotional?". "You're busy, God will surely understand." And yes, if you need to miss a day or two, that is fine. Just get back to it as soon as you possibly can so the devil can't continue to distract you. Stay strong in this four-week journey to strengthen your relationship with God and deepen your understanding in what He is calling you to achieve in your earthly days.

The bad news is that Satan will fight hard to derail you from your goals-especially if your goals are for God's glory. The good news is that we are not in this alone! We have our mighty Creator in our corner, rubbing our shoulders and helping us strategize against any temptation that comes our way. Seek the Lord daily, hourly, or maybe you will have days when you need his help every couple of minutes. He is there and ready to bestow His strength onto you. All you need to do is set your sight on Him and He will not fail you.

Before moving on to today's fitness routine, take a moment to re-read the Bible verse. What tempts you in your daily life? Acknowledge those temptations and meditate on the fact that you are stronger than all of them combined. There is a way around them, focus of finding it.

DAY TWO FITNESS ROUTINE

Please refer to the warm up on Page xv to prepare your body for today's exercise routine.

*PLANKS:

1. Start on your knees with either your hands or elbows directly under your shoulders. Bring your knees back past your hips and flex your toes.
Progression: Lift the knees off of the floor.
2. Engage your abdominals, visualizing hugging your spine so you feel it in your back, sides, and front.
3. Hold the plank position for 60 seconds. *This length of time is at your discretion. If you can't hold it that long yet, do what you can. You WILL eventually get there. If you can go longer than 60 seconds, hold the plank for as long as your body keeps proper form.

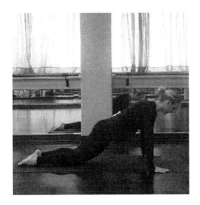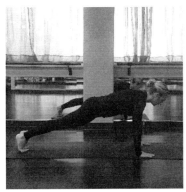

Progression Form

Plank Notes:

-Do not drop your head! Picture a fire under your face… you don't want to get burned!

-Make sure your body is in a nice diagonal line - no mountains with the hips lifted. No valleys with the hips dipped towards the floor.

-Create opposition with the floor. Bare down with either your hands or elbows.

-Last, but most important - KEEP YOUR ABDOMINALS TIGHTLY ENGAGED!

SIDELINE SERIES:

1. Lay on your right side with your right arm extended under the head. Stack your hips, knees, and ankles. Bring your legs in line with the rest of your body. Left hand on the floor in front of your chest to help with stability.
Modification: Bend your bottom leg to increase support and stability.

2. Engage your core. You should feel it in your front, sides, and back.
3. Take 2 counts to lift your top leg towards the ceiling.
4. Take 2 counts to lower the leg back down. Repeat 5-7 times.
5. Take 1 count to lift your leg towards the ceiling.
6. Take 1 count to lower your leg down. Repeat 8-10 times.
7. Lift your leg half-way up and, from the hip, move your leg in a circular motion (about the size of a soccer ball). Repeat 5-7 times.
8. Reverse the circular motion. Repeat 5-7 times.
   Repeat on the right side 2-3 times.
9. Repeat the series on the left side.

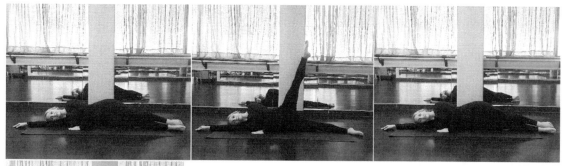

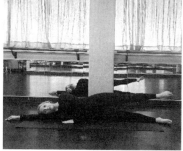

Sideline Series Notes:

-Pay attention to your top supporting arm. The goal is for your abdominals to do most of the stabilizing with the top arm assisting. If the top arm is getting tired, you are probably depending on it too much for stabilization.

-Work in your pain-free range of motion.

-When working in the circular motion, close your eyes and picture tracing the soccer ball sized circle. This visualization is a great distraction from the exercise itself.

FOREARM LEG EXTENSIONS:

1. Start by sitting up straight on the floor. Lean back to place your elbows on the floor under your shoulders, palms on the floor. Engage the core to length the spine. Bring both knees towards the chest.
2. Take 2 counts to extend your legs to the furthest point where the abdominals stay engaged. If you go too far out, the core will disengage.
3. Take 2 counts to bring the knees back towards the chest. Repeat 4-8 times.
4. Take 1 count to extend the legs.
5. Take 1 count to return the knees to the chest. Repeat 6-10 times.

Repeat series 2-4 times.

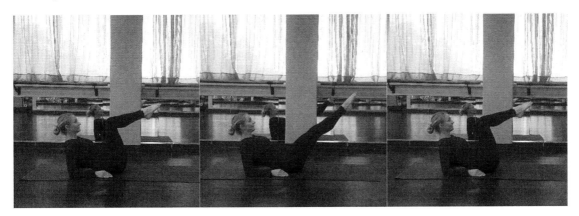

Forearm Leg Extension Notes:

-For weaker abdominals or tight hip flexors, refrain from fully extending the legs. Move in your comfortable range of motion.

-If you need support for your neck, place your head on the floor and keep the spine in contact with the floor.

-Press into the floor with your arms to keep from slumping into your shoulders. Keep your chest proud.

PIKE TRICEP PUSH-UPS:

1. Start in a plank position. Lift the hips towards the ceiling. The shoulders will shift back. *Modification: In a knee plank position, omit the hips lifting towards the ceiling.*

2. Bend at the elbows, allowing them to move towards the feet and not out to the sides.
3. Extend the arms.
4. Return to plank position. Repeat 5-10 times.

Rest and repeat the series as many times as you can while keeping proper form.

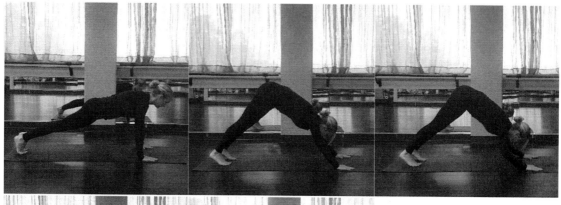

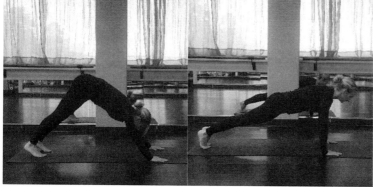

Pike Tricep Push-Ups:

-As the arms fatigue, the elbows will want to flare out to the sides. Keep your focus on the backwards movement of the arm bends.

-Be aware of dropping the head. Keep your eyes focused on the floor and not towards your feet.

Day Two done already? YES! Please reference Page xix for the cool down if needed.

Week Two – Day Three

Proverbs 25:28

> *Like a city whose walls are broken through is a person who lacks self-control.*

Let's start by understanding the purpose for a wall around a city. I think the most obvious reason for a wall is for protection. Without a barricade, a city is vulnerable to attacks and possibly being overtaken. If a city has a wall surrounding it, it must also have gates to allow and ultimately control what comes into the city and what goes out into the community. If the wall is not maintained and cared for, it will inevitably crumble. Similarly, if you and I lack self-control, we are as vulnerable to being captured by the enemy as a city with its walls broken to the ground.

Our success in achieving our goals and keeping our priorities depends on controlling our thoughts, desires, and actions. Personally, this is not something that comes naturally. I have always been quite the impulsive person. If I had a thought come to mind, almost immediately it would come out of my mouth. If I wanted a piece of German chocolate cake, I'd grab the biggest piece I could find without hesitation. As I got older, I grew wiser to the consequences of my lack of self-control. I would even go so far as to say I was embarrassed by it. Over time, I started to inspect my "wall"- my control over my earthly impulses. I found the weaknesses in its structure. With practice and God's help, I have learned to maintain and keep my "wall" strong. I'm not saying I never give into temptations. I still indulge in a piece of German chocolate cake from time to time, but I want my wall (my self-control) to strongly fortify my city (my soul).

Without self-control, we make Satan's job easier for him. The Bible verse simply means this: Your self-control keeps Satan from having victory and success in your life. Take the time to inspect your wall. Where are the weak spots? How good are your gates at controlling what comes into your life and what goes out into the community? Be honest with yourself. Once we acknowledge our temptations and weaknesses, we strip them of their power over us. With that, you will become a proper gate keeper of your spirit. When you can control your thoughts, impulses, and cravings, you control your success.

Every now and then, check in with yourself and do an inventory of temptations. They can change and evolve, so we need to stay on top of them to keep a truly fortified wall around our soul.

Before moving on to the exercises, search your "wall" for its weak spot. Addressing the temptations make them weaker and you stronger over them.

DAY THREE FITNESS ROUTINE

Please refer to the warm up on Page xv to prepare your body for today's exercise routine.

*BURPEES:

1. Stand with your legs wider than your body.
2. Bend the knees, and bring your hands to the floor directly under the shoulders.
3. Step back with the right leg to bring it directly behind the right hip. Repeat with the left leg. You will end up in a plank formation.
   Progression: Hop both legs out simultaneously into plank position and add a push up.
4. Step right leg up and then back to its starting position. Repeat with the left leg to end in a tuck position.
   Progression: Hop both legs back in at the same time.
5. Stand up.

Repeat as many times as you can without losing proper form.

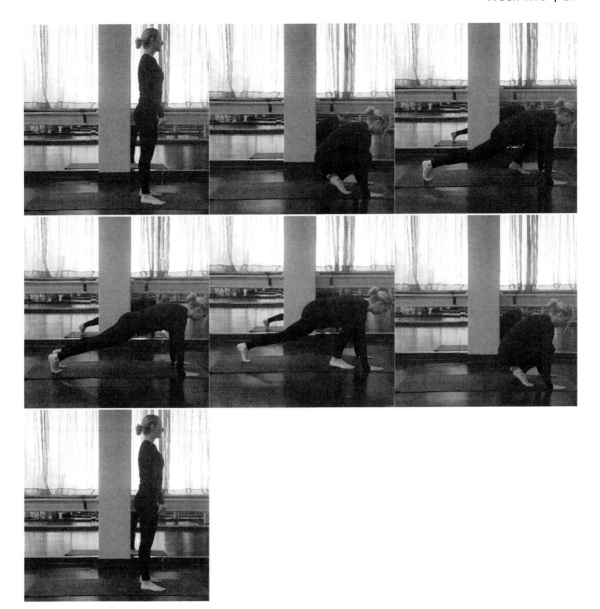

Burpee Notes:

-This can be a higher intensity exercise. If your body does not like this move for whatever reason, please replace this exercise with a previous one from earlier in the week.

-Keep track of the number of repetitions you complete. The number of reps completed will be your "Mile Marker."

-Go at your comfortable pace. Remember, you want to push yourself-not hurt yourself!

STANDING SIDE CRUNCHES:

1. Stand with your legs wide apart and turned out from the hips. Bend the knees to your lowest comfortable position. Roll the hips up towards the ribcage to neutralize your spine and then engage your abdominals in a baring down motion. Bring your hands behind your head with your elbows opened to the sides.
   Progression: Slightly lean back to further engage abdominals. Modification: Slightly lean forward to ease abdominal engagement.
2. At your own pace, crunch laterally to the right. Feel the side abdominals (the obliques) contract.
3. Using the left side obliques, lift the torso to return directly over hips.
4. Repeat on the right side 20-40 times.
5. Repeat the series crunching to the left 20-40 times.

   Rest and repeat the series 2-3 times.

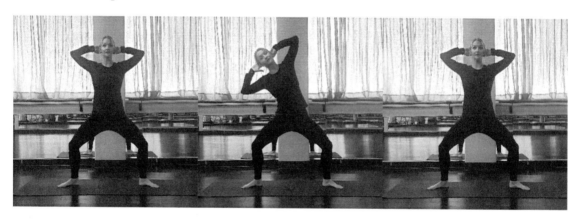

Standing Side Crunch Notes:

-The goal of this exercise is to get the elbows as close as you can to your thighs without lowering your arms.

-Go at your own comfortable pace and range of motion.

-Stay low in your legs to engage the glutes and quadriceps.

-It is important to keep the abdominals tight to support the lateral flexion of the spine.

BEAST MODE SERIES: (IT IS NOT AS SCARY AS IT SOUNDS!)

1. Start on the floor on all fours with your hands or elbows under your shoulders. Place your knees directly under your hips. Engage the core to position the spine straight (not dipping towards the floor). Extend your head and neck.
2. Lift your knees an inch to hover over the floor. Hold for 10 seconds.
3. Return knees to the floor.
4. Return the knees to the hover position.
5. Tap the floor with your knees and then return to the hover. Keep the movement small. Repeat 10 times and stretch if needed.
6. Return to hover position.
7. Take a small step to the right with the right foot.
8. Take a small step to the left with the left foot.
9. Return the right foot in line with the body.
10. Return the left foot in line with the body. Repeat 3-6 times

    Repeat series 1-3 times.

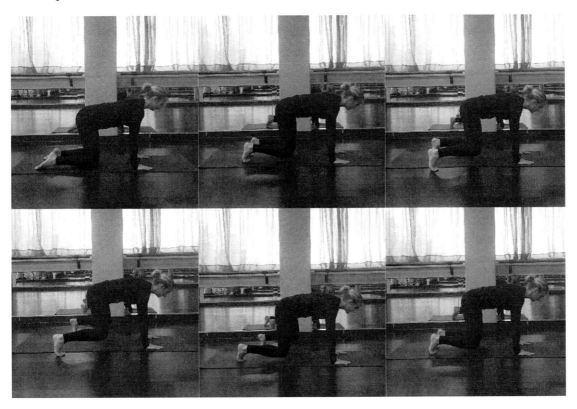

Beast Mode Notes:

-Stretch throughout the series as needed.

-If you feel tension in your wrists, lower onto your elbows.

-Every now and then glance down at your knees, make sure the hover is no more than an inch. Besides that, don't drop your head.

-This is a full body exercise. Your upper body and core are engaged for support and your lower body engages during the movement. Learn to love the burn!

"U" BRIDGES:

1. Lay on your back and place your feet flat on the floor with your ankles under your knees, your legs hip distant apart. To imprint your spine onto the floor, roll your hips up towards the ribcage and engage the abdominals to press the spine into the floor. Place your arms by your sides. Engage your glutes (your bottom) to lift the hips towards the ceiling.
    Modification: If your knees don't allow for that range of motion, bring your feet forward until you find a comfortable position.
    Progression: Lift the heels off of the floor and press the balls of your feet down. Lift arms towards ceiling.
2. Imagine a "U" under your seat. Relax the glutes to lower the hips. Trace up the right side of the "U" and engage only the right glute muscle. The right hip will be higher than the left.
3. Relax the glutes and then trace up the left side of the "U." Engage solely the left glute muscle and allow the left hip to rise higher than the right hip. This motion can be as large or small as you need. The larger the "U," the more effective. Repeat 10-15 times holding at the top right of your last repetition.
4. At the top right of your "U," slightly relax the contraction of the right glute muscle then quickly reengage the glute for a pulsing motion. Repeat the pulses about 20-30 times.
5. Relax the muscles to travel to the top left of the "U." Repeat the pulses on the left side 20-30 times.

    Repeat the series 2-3 times.

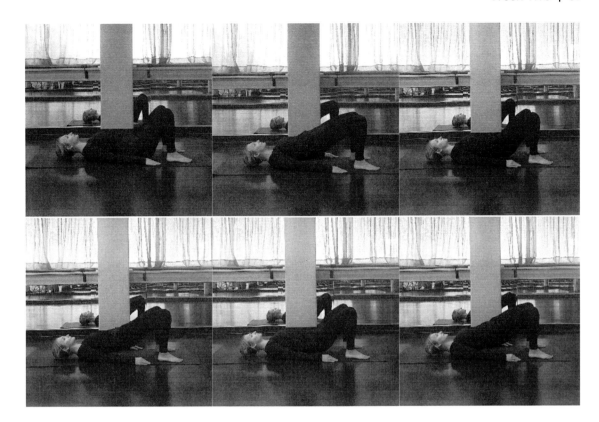

"U" Bridge Notes:

-To maximize this exercise, pay close attention to the contraction vs. relaxation of the glutes. When you're at the top of your bridge, your glutes are tight; when you lower to the floor, there is no contraction at all.

-You should never feel pressure in the back of your neck. If you do, lower your hips.

-Make sure you engage only one side of the bottom at a time.

Day Three is completed. Excellent! Don't forget your cool down.

Week Two – Day Four

Galatians 5:16-17

> *"So I say, walk by the Spirit, and you will not gratify the desires of the flesh. For the flesh desires what is contrary to the Spirit, and the Spirit what is contrary to the flesh. They are in conflict with each other, so that you are not to do whatever you want."*

What is the difference between self-control and self-discipline? Why must we have both? In 2 Timothy, we saw that self-discipline is given to us by God. In 1 Corinthians, we learned that there will always be temptations, but there is also always a way out provided by God. (We just need to have the awareness and self-control to follow that path.) In yesterday's passage, it became clear that without self-control we will fail against our earthly urges. In today's reading, we learn that we must have both self-control and self-discipline.

We need to control the desires of our flesh and use the discipline gifted to us in order to pursue the desires of the Holy Spirit. With self-control, we dampen the cravings and sometimes sinful urges of the flesh. This is mastered with time and repetitive practice. The use of self-discipline helps us put into action the things we know we should do.

The Spirit desires the opposite of our earthly vessels, but it is our earthly vessels that have to perform the duties of the Spirit. That is enough to make your head spin! Thank the Lord that He gave us the power, strength, and self-discipline we need in order to satisfy the Spirit. Control your impulses and use discipline in your actions.

Before moving on to today's fitness routine, think of a time you found yourself fighting the battle between the desires of the Spirit and the flesh. Who won? The Spirit or the flesh? What did you learn from that experience?

DAY FOUR FITNESS ROUTINE- HAND WEIGHTS

Please refer to the warm up on Page xv to prepare your body for today's exercise routine.

-Start with heavier weights and feel free to move to a lighter weight at any point. Weights are not required but recommended to maximize your results.

TRADITIONAL BICEP CURLS:

1. Standing with your legs hip distant apart, bring your arms by your sides with the palms facing front. Bring your arms slightly in front of your body.
   Progression: Lift your arms shoulder height.
   Place an imaginary table under your elbows so they don't lower.
2. Flexing at the elbows, bring your palms towards your shoulders. Give your biceps a good tight flex. Work in your comfortable full range of motion.
3. Extend your arms and reach long in front. Repeat 7-10 times.
4. Again, flex at the elbows to bring the palms in towards the shoulders but stop half way. Hands will be in line with the elbows.
5. Fully extend the arms back out. Repeat 10-15 times.

   Repeat series 2-3 times.

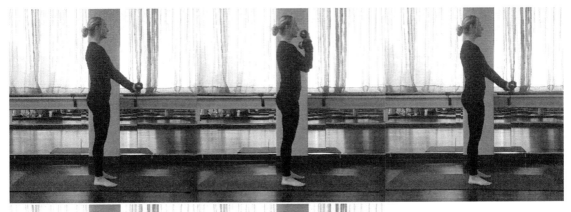

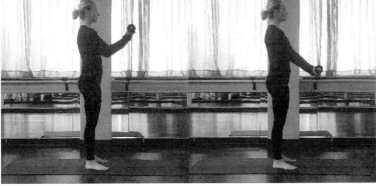

Bicep Curl Notes:
-Keep the spine tall and shoulders down; reach the ears in opposition from the shoulders.
-Stay strong in the wrists so the weights don't cause the wrist to bend.

ROWS:

1. Stand with your ankles directly under your hips. Bend your knees and hinge forward from the hips. Slightly tilt the pelvis forward and engage the abdominals. Roll the shoulders back/around/and down; chest is proud. Reach the shoulders low down the spine. The neck is long. Allow your eyes to focus on the floor a few feet in front of you to keep your neck in proper position.
2. Bring your arms under the shoulders with your palms facing your body.
3. Lift the arms up and back to bring the shoulder blades towards the spine.
4. Return to starting position. Repeat 5-10 times.
5. Rotate the arms so that the palms are facing each other. Lift the elbows up and bring the shoulder blades towards the spine. Keep the elbows close to the torso. Repeat 5-10 times.

    Repeat series 2-3 times.

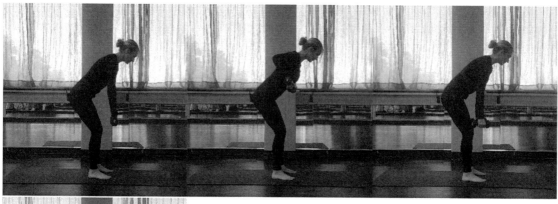

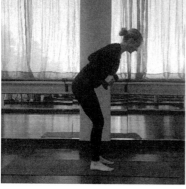

Row Notes:

-Work in your pain-free range of motion.

-Keep abdominals engaged to support the spine during the twisting motion.

-If tension builds up in the neck, check your position. Are your shoulders slowly creeping up? Is your head dropping?

TRICEP LIFTS:

1. Return to your hinge position. Stand with your ankles directly under your hips. Bend your knees and hinge forward from the hips. Slightly tilt the pelvis forward and engage the abdominals. Roll the shoulders back/around/and down; chest is proud. Reach the shoulders low down the spine. The neck is long.
2. Extend the arms towards the floor directly under the shoulders, palms facing each other.
3. Take 2 counts to lift the arms behind to your highest comfortable point.
4. Take 2 counts to lower the arms to starting position. Repeat 5-10 times.
5. Take 2 counts to lift just the right arm behind you.
6. Take 2 counts to return the right arm down. Repeat 5-10 times.
7. Repeat on the left side 5-10 times.

    Repeat series 2-3 times.

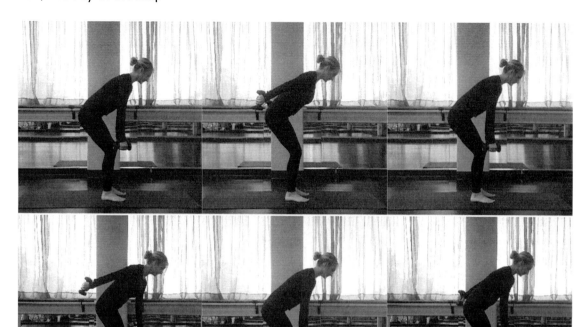

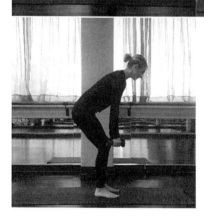

Tricep Lift Notes:

-Work in your pain-free range of motion.

-If you need to go slower, please do so.

-If tension builds up in the neck, check your position. Are your shoulders slowly creeping up? Is your head dropping?

-Keep your core engaged to support the hinged spine.

-Keep the body weight in the back of the feet. Try wiggling your toes to check for this.

-Be cautious not to allow the arms to swing past the shoulders as you lower them.

LATERAL ARM LIFTS:

1. Stand with your heels together and your toes apart. Engage the core and depress the shoulder down the spine. Reach the top of your head towards the ceiling. Arms are down by your side with palms in towards your body.
2. Take 2 counts to lift your arms to the side to shoulder height.
   Modification: For shoulder pain, lift to your highest pain-free point.
3. Take 2 counts to lower the arms back to your sides. Repeat 5-10 times.
4. Repeat lifting only the right arm 5-10 times.
5. Repeat lifting on the left side 5-10 times.

   Repeat series 2-3 times.

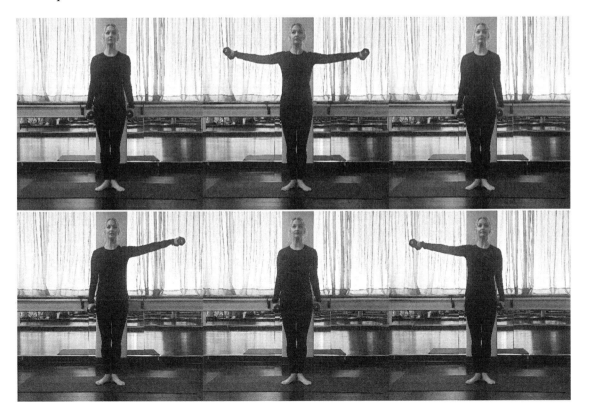

Lateral Arm Lift Notes:

-Work in your pain-free range.

-Control the motion on the way down. Don't let gravity pull the arm down.

If it doesn't challenge you, it doesn't change you! Remember to cool down.

Week Two – Day Five

1 Corinthians 9:25-26

> *"Everyone who competes in the games goes into strict training. They do it to get a crown that will not last, but we do it to get a crown that will last forever. Therefore I do not run like someone running aimlessly; I do not fight like a boxer beating at the air."*

It doesn't matter what the goal is. Whether it is a spiritual or physical goal, to achieve it, takes three things: self-control, self-discipline, and a plan. In this verse, Paul warns us about reckless ambitions. Like an athlete training for a competition, we, as Christians, must also put in the daily effort. Our salvation doesn't depend on it, thank you Jesus, but we are called to live a life showing God's grace and constantly striving to grow in our faith.

What is your goal and how are you going to make it a reality? Do you want to grow closer in your relationship with the Lord? Do you want a stronger prayer life? Is there a physical objective you're aiming for? For your plan to succeed it needs to be S.M.A.R.T.!

S- Specific. Think about the details. The more details you have, the smoother the plan is likely to go.

M- Measurable. Give yourself markers along the way so you know when you're on the right track.

A- Attainable. Be honest with yourself. Know your strengths and weaknesses before you start. Of course you want to push yourself, but you don't want to set yourself up for failure.

R- Realistic. Have you tried this before? What did you learn from your success/failure? How can you adapt and grow in this plan?

T- Timely. Give yourself a timeline. When can you expect to be half-way there? When will you complete your plan? Avoid boredom and abandoning your goal by shortening the timeline while still being realistic.

During our time here on earth, we will receive rewards for our efforts. Although, they might make us happy, it is important to realize that our true reward waits for us in heaven. It is inevitable; you will reap the physical benefits from the hard work you put into having a *Body of Worship*. Keep your heavenly goal at the forefront. With your healthier body, you are able to accomplish more of what the Lord is calling you to do. And that is more satisfying than anything else you can imagine.

Read the verse above once more. Do your actions have purpose or are you a boxer beating at the air? Think of your earthly and spiritual goals. What is your S.M.A.R.T. plan to achieve them?

DAY FIVE FITNESS ROUTINE

Please refer to the warm up on Page xv to prepare your body for today's exercise routine.

CALF RAISES:

1. If needed, stand close to something that can help you balance, a chair for example. With your heels together and toes apart, stretch the spine upwards and engage your abdominals in a baring down motion.
2. Lift the heels off of the floor engaging your calf muscles. Feel the weight dispersed evenly amongst the balls of your feet and all ten toes.
3. Slowly, with control, lower the heels to the floor. Resist the temptation to rock back to your heels. Repeat 8 times.
4. Lift your heels and then only lower half-way down to the floor. Repeat 8 times.
5. Lift your heels and pulse just an inch or so in a bouncing motion. Continue for a count of 16.

Repeat series 2-3 times.

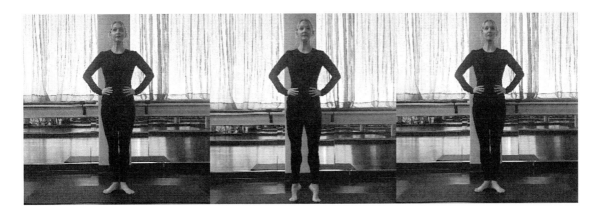

Calf Raise Notes:

-Feel free to take a break when needed and roll the ankle. This exercise will strengthen both the muscle and joint. Honor your body when it needs a break!

-This can also be done in a parallel position with the toes in front of the heels.

*BICYCLE OBLIQUE CRUNCHES:

1. Lay on your back and bring both legs to table top position. Spread out your fingertips, cradle the back of your head, and bring the elbows away from the face. Lift your head and shoulder blades from the floor. Imprint your spine onto the floor.
2. Extend your right leg to the ceiling and lower it to a comfortable level where the spine is still in contact with the floor.
   Modification: Keep both legs bent with feet flat on the floor.
3. Rotate the upper body bringing the right shoulder towards the left knee. Hold for a count of 4.
4. Switch sides. Return the right leg to table top and extend the left leg in front. Rotate the upper body bringing the left shoulder towards the right knee. Hold for a count of 4. Repeat at this pace 4-8 times on each side.
5. Continue the same movement holding the crunch for 2 counts on each side. Repeat 6-10 times on each side.
6. Continue the bicycle motion speeding up the crunch hold for 1 count on each side. Repeat 8-12 times on each side.

*Progression: *Move through the bicycle motion as fast as you can while keeping good form. Continue the "cardio cycle" for as long as you can. Keep track of your time and use this progression as a "Mile Marker."*

Repeat series 1-3 times.

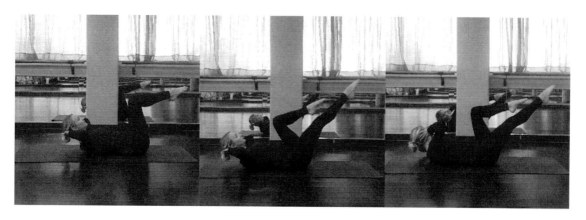

Bicycle Oblique Crunch Notes:

-Allow your elbows to be seen in your peripheral vision. If they are too wide, it can cause straining in the neck and shoulders. If the elbows are too close to the face, you're probably pulling on the neck causing unnecessary tension.

-If your hips start to feel tight, don't fully extend your legs.

-Make sure it's the shoulder and not the elbow that is aiming towards the knee. This will ensure proper oblique engagement.

-Allow the weight of your head to fully rest in your hands to minimize neck discomfort.

ALL 4'S LEG LIFTS:

1. Begin on all fours. Your hands or elbows under your shoulders and your knees under your hips. Engage the abdominals to keep the spine straight and not bending towards the floor. Extend the head and neck away from the shoulders.
2. Keeping the right leg bent, take 2 counts to lift the right knee to the side to your comfortable highest position.
3. Take 2 counts to return the knee under the hip. (Repeat 5-8 times hold at the top of your last repetition)

4. Working in the circumduction of the hip socket, move the leg in a circular motion as if you are tracing a soccer ball with your knee. Complete 5-10 circles.
5. Reverse the circle and complete 5-10 more.
6. Lower the knee to the floor under the hip. Lower the tailbone towards the heels and stretch in "Child's Pose."
7. Return to all fours and repeat series on left side.

Repeat series 2-3 times.

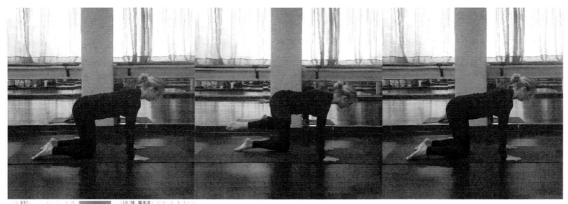

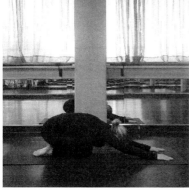

All 4's Leg Lift Notes:

-If your wrists start to fatigue, lower to your elbows.

-Work in your pain-free range. The height of the leg is up to you.

-Resist the temptation to lean to one side by keeping your weight centered.

-Don't drop your head.

LEG LIFTS:

1. Still lying on your back, bring your legs one at a time to table top position.
2. Roll the hips up towards the ribcage until the spine is fully on the floor.
3. Engage the abdominals to the point of pressing the spine deeply into the floor.
4. Extend your legs to the ceiling and lower the legs forward. Your spine should still be pressed firmly down by the abdominals.
   Modification: Bend at the knees to shorten the lever. If you need support for your low back, place your hands under your tailbone. For more stability, cross at the ankles.
   Progression: Turn out from the hips and press your heels together until you feel your inner thighs engage.
5. Taking four counts, slowly lift your legs back over the hips.
6. Again, for four counts, lower the legs forward stopping before the low back lifts off of the floor. Repeat 5-10 times, holding with your legs lifted after the last repetition.
7. Lower the legs in two counts.
8. Taking two counts, lift the legs to return over the hips. Repeat 5-10 times, holding your legs in the lifted position at the end.
9. Speed up the motion to one count down, and one count up. Please shorten your range of motion to protect your hip joints and back. Repeat 10-15 times.

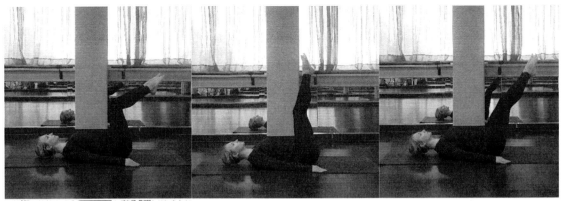

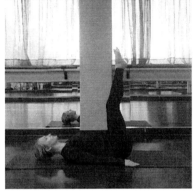

Leg Lift Notes:

-Make sure you don't hold your breath. Continue breathing! Inhale as you lower the legs, and exhale as you lift them.

-If you start to feel your hips gripping or getting tight, bend your knees and shorten your range of motion.

-Don't press your arms down into the floor. Make that your abs' job.

-Your spine naturally curves, so you'll need to keep your abdominals engaged to keep your spine straight… Stay focused. If you feel your spine starting to come off of the floor, don't lower your legs so far down.

Day 5 complete – Congrats. Keep up the good work!

Week Two – Day Six

Proverbs 16:32

> *"Better a patient person than a warrior, one with self-control than one who takes a city."*

The imagery of an angry and hasty warrior storming a city's gate floods my mind when I read this passage. I don't know about you, but I don't want to resemble that person- not with my family, not in my daily life, and definitely not in my spiritual journey. In this passage, the Lord is telling us to be patient. We all know it is important to be patient with others, but how about with ourselves? We are our own worst critics. We bestow kindness and grace to others but can be so hard on ourselves. This needs to change. I believe that so strongly that I dedicated next week's chapter to self-love and renewal.

Any transformation takes time, especially when it comes to living a healthier lifestyle. There will be so many changes that will take place in your life that setbacks will be a sure thing. Being prepared for the occasional lapse will allow you to be patient and forgiving towards yourself.

Once again, the scripture is stressing the importance of self-control. Controlling one's impulses is vital to success in any venture. Today, think about controlling your urge to pick yourself apart and beat yourself down when setbacks occur. A setback does not mean you are weak. It simply means you are human. If you come across an exercise or activity that is not conducive to your body's capabilities, shrug it off and replace it with one of your favorites. Remember that this program is designed for you to learn how to honor your body; not just in what it can do, but also in listening to its limitations.

Before you move on to today's fitness routine, read the verse again. Think of a time when you were patient with another person. It probably was not the easiest thing you've ever done, but you knew it was necessary. Remember that feeling the next time you need to be patient with yourself.

DAY SIX FITNESS ROUTINE

Please refer to Page xv for your warm up.

KNEE HUGS:

1. Lay on your back with your legs extended on the floor hip distance apart and your arms out to the sides with your palms facing the ceiling.
2. Take 4 counts to lift your head and shoulder blades from the floor. At the same time, bring your knees towards your chest. Hug your arms around your shins. Hold for a single count.
   Modification: Leave your head and shoulder blades on the floor.
3. Simultaneously, take 4 counts to lower the legs and upper body to the floor. Allow the spine to lift from the floor when you're completely back down. Repeat 4-6 times.
4. Repeat the series using a quicker pace at 2 counts to rise and 2 counts to lower. Repeat 6-8 times.

   Repeat series 2-3 times.

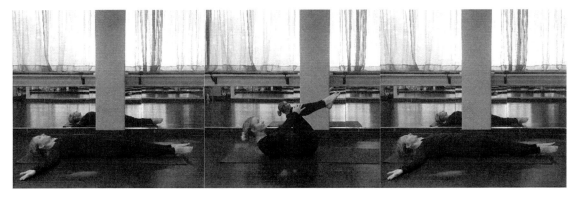

Knee Hug Notes:

-Allow the body to completely relax when you come back down to the floor. Then re-contract the muscles as you start your next repetition.

-Keep the legs moving together. As you fatigue, the legs will want to start moving at separate times.

-If your neck gets tired, embrace the modification.

*TRICEP PUSH-UPS:

1. Starting on all fours, place your hands directly under the shoulders with the fingers pointing forward. Bring your knees back past your hips. Engage the core so the spine does not dip towards the floor. Your neck is long.
   Progression: Lift the knees from the floor into a full push-up position.

2. Taking 3 counts, bend at the elbows allowing the arms to brush the sides of your body as your torso lowers towards the floor.
3. Take a single count to extend the arms to return to starting position. Repeat 4-6 times.
4. Reverse the counts. Take 1 count to lower the body and 3 counts to extend at the elbow to raise the body. Repeat 4-6 times.
5. Continue the same motion, taking 1 count down and 1 count to come up. Repeat as many times as you can while keeping proper form.

   Repeat series 1-3 times.

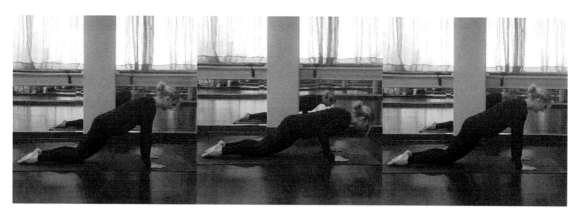

Tricep Push-up Notes:

-*Due to the difficulty level of this exercise, the number of repetitions you are able to complete is your "Mile Marker."*

-*Do not drop your head towards the floor.*

-*Keep the abdominals engaged to support the spine.*

-*Tell yourself to squeeze your ribs with your elbows. This will help you keep the arms close to the body.*

-*Allow the elbows to bend in such a way that they are "pointing" in the direction of your toes.*

SPINAL EXTENSION WITH LEG WORK:

1. Lay on your stomach with your hands stacked under your forehead and legs fully extended, reaching towards the wall behind you. Open your legs to a comfortable wider position.
2. Lift your legs from the floor.

3. Take a single count to bring your legs together.
4. Take a single count to return them to the wide position. Repeat 5-10 times and hold wide after your last repetition.
5. Take 2 counts to lower the legs to the floor.
6. Take 2 counts to lift the legs back up. Repeat 5-10 times.

Repeat series 2-4 times.

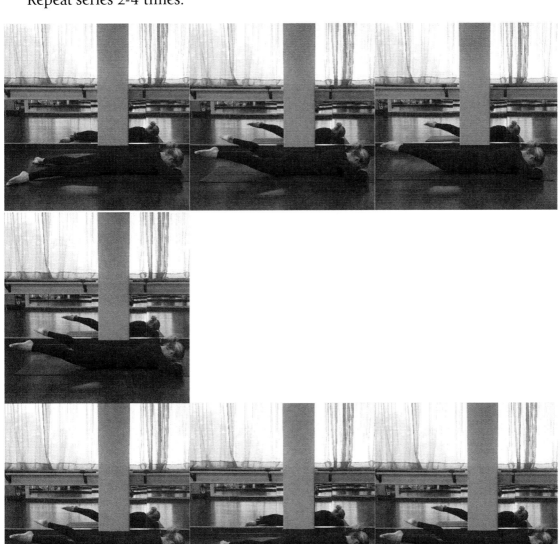

Spinal Extension with Leg Work Notes:

-If you're pointing your toes and reaching too hard behind you in your legs, you might experience muscle cramps. If this occurs, flex your feet and extend through the heels rather the toes.

-Engage the abdominals to keep the hips from pressing too hard into the floor.

HIP TWIST PLANKS:

1. Start on the floor with either your hands or elbows directly under your shoulders. Bring your knees past your hips and flex your toes.
   Progression: Lift the knees off of the floor.
2. Engage your abdominals, visualizing hugging your spine so you feel it in your back, sides, and front.
3. Keeping abdominals engaged, twist the right hip towards the floor.
4. Lower the right hip towards the floor to a comfortable position.
   Modification: Omit the hip dip after the twist.
5. Lift the right hip and square both hips to the floor.
6. Repeat on the left side.
7. Repeat the twisting motion on both sides 4-6 times.

   Rest if needed and repeat the series again 2-3 times.

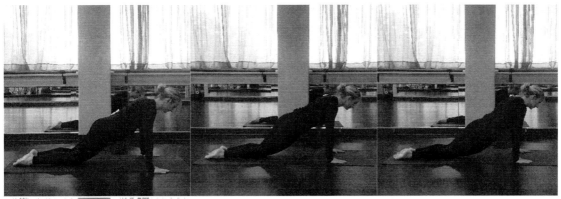

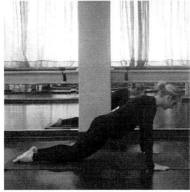

Hip Twist Plank Notes:

-It helps to speak or think to yourself, "Twist, Dip, Lift, Come Center."

-As you lower the hip towards the floor, the abdominals will want to disengage. Be aware of this and keep them tight!

-Go at your own pace and range of motion.

-Keep your head lifted.

Great Work! You are officially half-way through the program. I'm so proud of you!

WEEK THREE

A Body of Worship is renewed and has self-love.

Week Three – Day One

Romans 12:2

> *"Do not conform to the pattern of this world, but be transformed by the renewing of your mind. Then you will be able to test and approve what God's will is – his good, pleasing, and perfect will."*

One of my favorite sayings is "The body achieves what the mind believes." So many times we have preconceived notions of our body's capabilities and limitations. Today, I want to bring your attention to the consequences of any negativity you may have towards yourself. How many times have you avoided doing something simply by saying, "Oh, there is no way I could do that!"? That very thought, that lie that Satan places in our heads, has kept us in the comfort zone too many times. Some of us do have handicaps and physical limitations that can stop us, but that's not what I'm talking about in this instance; it is the paralyzing thoughts that tell you failure is inevitable, that you're not capable, or why even bother. Those are the enemy's whispers. Do you think Satan wants us stronger, healthier, more capable, and full of confidence? He sure does not.

Transform your thoughts. Protect yourself from the lies that have kept you from stepping out of the comfort zone. You are capable of so much and when you renew your mind to believe that, you are allowing God to use you for His good, perfect, and pleasing plans. Challenge yourself physically and spiritually in the coming days to do something outside that comfort zone. Break down the walls the negative thoughts have built. Love yourself enough to say, "I have never done that. Let me try." You just might surprise yourself.

Before moving onto the exercises, read the verse one more time. Start the process of renewing your mind today. Remove the negative preconceived thoughts about your capabilities. You are a strong person that has God-given talents to be used here on earth. When you seek God's will for your life and use the skills He has planted in you, you are unstoppable.

DAY ONE FITNESS ROUTINE

Please refer to Page xv to warm up your body before today's exercises.

SQUATS:

1. Begin by standing with your legs a little wider than your hips and hands pressed together in front of the chest in prayer position with your elbows lifted. Engage core.
2. Hinge forward from the hips and bend the knees to bring your seat towards the floor.
3. Extend your legs and bring your torso upright. Repeat 10-15 times.
4. Bend the knees and hinge forward into your squat position. Hold.
5. Lower the seat down about six inches and quickly return to starting position. Keep the weight in your heels. Repeat 20-30 times.

Repeat series 2-4 times.

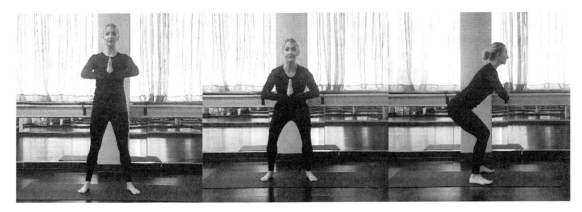

Squat Notes:

-Always move in your pain-free range.

-Keep the weight in your heels to activate the back of the body.

-Keep the core engaged, ribs and naval pulled in towards the spine, to support the spinal movement.

-Press your hands together and keep the elbows lifted to activate the chest and the shoulders.

LEG LIFT PUSH-UPS:

1. Begin on all fours with hands under the shoulders and knees under the hips. Engage core. Bring the knees back further past the hips. Extend the right leg to the side with the toes touching the floor.
2. Bend the elbows to lower the chest towards the floor. Simultaneously, as you lower the upper body, lift the right leg to the ceiling.
3. Extend the arms and lower the leg back to starting position. Repeat 5-10 times.
4. Repeat lifting the left leg 5-10 times.

   Rest and repeat the series 2-3 times.

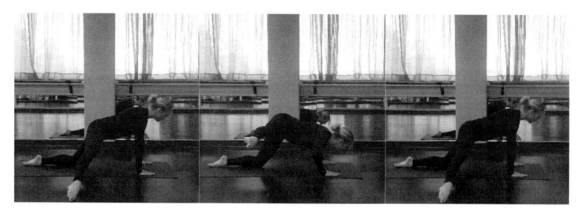

Leg Lift Push-up Notes:

-Be cautious not to drop the head and abdominals towards the floor.

-Lift the legs in your comfortable range of motion.

CRUNCH ENDURANCE SERIES:

1. Begin by lying on your back with your feet flat on the floor. Spread out your fingers and cradle the back of your head. Lift your head and shoulder blades from the floor.
2. Contract the abdominals to lift the shoulder blades a little higher.
3. Slightly release to return to starting position. Repeat 8-15 times.
4. Bring the right leg to table top position; your knee over the hips and the shin parallel to the floor. Hold the leg in position and complete 8-15 crunches.
5. Bring the left leg to table top to match the right leg. Complete 8-15 crunches.
6. Extend both legs towards the ceiling. Complete 8-15 crunches.

7. Open legs into straddle stretch and complete 8-15 crunches.
8. Bring legs back together towards the ceiling and complete 8-15 crunches.
9. Bring both legs to table top position and complete 8-15 crunches.
10. Place right foot on the floor keeping the left leg in table top position. Complete 8-15 crunches.
11. Place both feet onto the floor and complete your last round of 8-15 crunches.

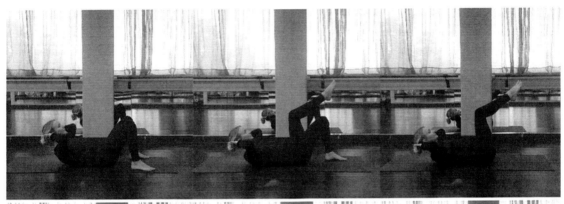

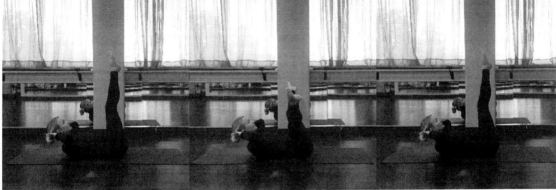

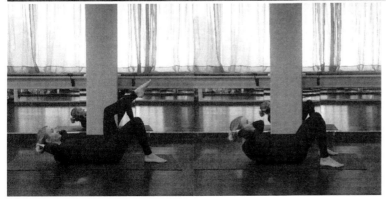

Crunch Notes:

-Keep your elbows in your peripheral vision. If the elbows come too close to your head, you're more likely to be pulling your head forward creating strain in your neck. If your elbows move outside your peripheral vision, strain is likely to occur in the chest and shoulders.

-If tension occurs in your neck, place your head on the floor and rest for a few seconds.

-This is a longer series, so if you need to take a break, go for it. Just get back where you started.

-Allow the weight of your head to rest in your spread out finger tips to help release tension in neck.

CRISS-CROSS LEG LIFTS:

1. Lying on your back, place your hands under your tailbone, and bring your toes up to the ceiling. Cross at the ankles and soften your knees. Imprint your spine onto the floor and fully engage abdominals.
    Progression: Place your hands on the floor by your sides. Palms down.
2. As you lower your legs towards the floor in front of you, uncross your ankles and re-cross (about 3-4 times). Don't allow the spine to leave the floor. If your spine does want to pop up, don't lower your legs as much.
3. As you lift your legs back towards the ceiling, crisscross your ankles again about 3-4 times. Repeat 5-10 times.

    Rest if needed and repeat the series again 2-3 times.

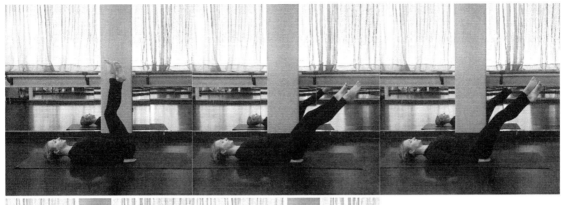

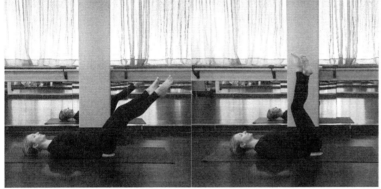

Criss-Cross Leg Lift Notes:

-Keep your knees slightly bent and if you feel your hips becoming tight, bend your knees even more.

-Don't forget to breathe! Exhale as your legs lower and inhale as your legs lift.

Your first day of your third week was a success. Great work! Don't forget to cool down.

Week Three – Day Two

Psalm 139:14

> *"I praise you because I am fearfully and wonderfully made; your works are wonderful, I know that full well."*

Your body is amazing. Did you know that in just one minute:

- the heart on average pumps 1.5 gallons of blood?
- the kidneys can clean 1.2 liters of blood?
- the brain processes 600 million particles of visual information?
- 12,000,000,000,000,000 signals are sent through nerve impulses in the brain?
- collectively your hair grows 1.1 inch? (rd.com) … and the list goes on!

If we knew exactly what goes on in our physical bodies and what all they are capable of doing, the sense of awe would be overwhelming. God's design of the human body is nothing short of a masterpiece.

He did not make a single mistake when He personally designed you! If you are eating healthy and are exercising regularly, then you look just as the Lord intended. We often compare ourselves with others. When we feel like we come up short, intimidation, lack of self-worth, and maybe even depression can take over. As a society, we need to remember that "healthy" looks different of everybody. You can look on social media today and quickly witness people taking their physical appearance to extremes. Whether it is the body builder or the fitness model, their outward appearance does not necessarily translate into their inward appearance – health wise, mentally, or spiritually.

You know you are a one-of-a-kind, hand-made, work of art, so there is no need to compare yourself with anyone. You, dear friend, are wonderfully made by the Almighty Father! Take a moment and let that sink in. Take a moment to thank God for your attributes and characteristics. If you're struggling with body image issues, ask the Lord to show you what He sees in you. It is amazing!

Before moving on to the exercise portion for today, take a moment to read the Bible verse again. Allow God to show you how wonderful you are. Ask the Lord to allow you to be able to see yourself through His eyes. God took His time to know you and create all the details that make you "you." There is nothing more comforting than that!

DAY TWO FITNESS ROUTINE

Today is a big "Mile Marker" day!

Please refer to Page xv for your warm up if needed.

*PLANKS / MOUNTAIN CLIMBERS:

1. Start on the floor with either your hands or elbows directly under your shoulders. Bring your knees past your hips and flex your toes. Lift your knees off of the floor.
   Modification: Keep your knees on the floor.
2. Engage your abdominals, visualize hugging your spine so you feel it in your back, sides, and front.
3. Hold the plank position for 60 seconds. *This length of time is at your discretion. If you can't hold for that long yet, do what you can. You WILL eventually get there. If you can go longer than 60 seconds, hold the plank for as long as your body keeps proper form.
4. Rest and, if able, reset into a full plank starting position for Mountain Climbers.
5. Slowly, bring your right knee towards your chest without moving your torso.
6. At the same slow pace, return the leg to plank.
7. Repeat on the left side.

Repeat on both sides as many times as you can while keeping proper form.

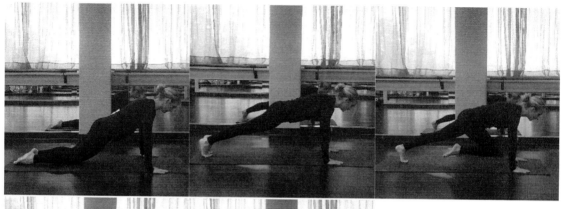

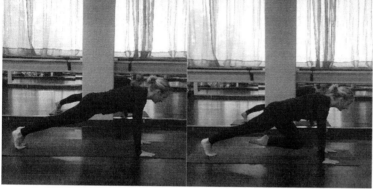

Plank & Mountain Climber Notes:

-*Do not drop your head. Picture a fire under your face and you don't want to get burned!*

-*Make sure your body is in a nice diagonal line…. No mountains with the hips lifted. No valleys with the hips dipped towards the floor.*

-*Create opposition with the floor. Bare down with either your hands or elbows.*

-*During the Mountain Climbers, if you'd like to incorporate some cardio into your routine, you may speed up the pace of that movement as long as you keep proper form.*

-*Mountain Climbers can be done in knee plank form as well.*

-*Lastly, but most important - KEEP YOUR ABDOMINALS TIGHTLY ENGAGED!*

*BICYCLE OBLIQUE CRUNCHES:

1. Lay on your back and bring both legs to table top position. Spread out your fingertips, cradle the back of your head, and bring the elbows away from the face. Lift your head and shoulder blades from the floor. Imprint your spine onto the floor.
2. Extend your right leg to the ceiling and lower it to a comfortable level where the spine is still in contact with the floor.
   Modification: Keep both legs bent with feet flat on the floor.
3. Rotate the upper body bringing the right shoulder towards the left knee. Hold for a count of 4.
4. Switch sides. Return the right leg to table top and extend the left leg in front. Rotate the upper body bringing the left shoulder towards the right knee. Hold for a count of 4. Repeat at this pace 4-8 times on each side.
5. Continue the same movement holding the crunch for 2 counts on each side. Repeat 6-10 times on each side.
6. Continue the bicycle motion speeding up the crunch hold for 1 count on each side. Repeat 8-12 times on each side.
   *Progression: *Move through the bicycle motion as fast as you can while keeping good form. Continue the "cardio cycle" for as long as you can. Keep track of your time and use this progression as a "Mile Marker."*

Repeat series 1-3 times.

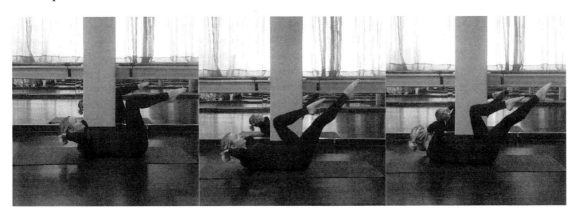

Bicycle Oblique Crunch Notes:

-Allow your elbows to be seen in your peripheral vision. If they are too wide, it can cause straining in the neck and shoulders. If they are too close to the face, you're probably pulling on the neck causing unnecessary tension.

-If your hips start to feel tight, don't fully extend your legs.

-Make sure it's the shoulder, and not the elbow, that is aiming towards the knee. This will ensure proper oblique engagement.

-Allow the weight of your head to fully rest in your hands to minimize neck discomfort.

BALANCE SERIES:

1. Stand with your heels together and your toes apart. Engage the core and stretch the spine tall towards the ceiling. Hands on your hips. If you know balance is not your strong suit, grab a chair or another prop to assist you.
2. Draw your right toes up the left leg. Open at the hip to the bring knee more towards the right. Engage your glutes.
   Progression: Take the toe away from the standing leg.
3. Slowly bring the knee in front of the hip. Moving at your own comfortable pace.
4. Slowly bring the knee back open to the starting position. Repeat 4-6 times.
5. Slowly extend and bend the leg. Repeat 4-6 times.
6. Moving at a faster pace if possible, continue to extend and bend the leg. Repeat the smaller movement 15-20 times.
7. Repeat series with left leg.

   Repeat series 1-2 times.

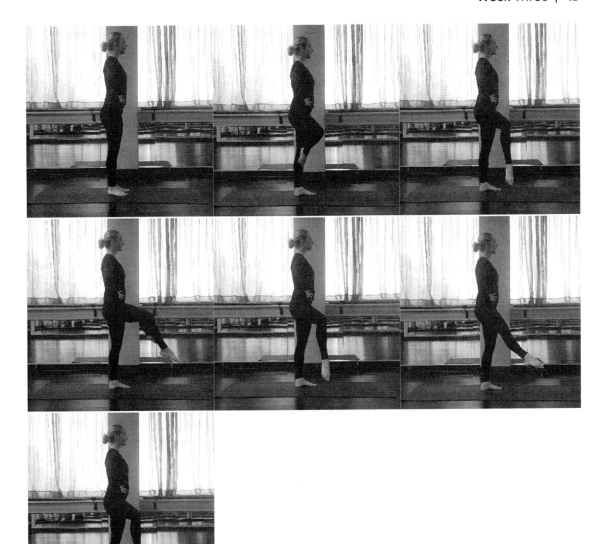

Balance Series Notes:

-If you need to take a quick break, go for it. Just get right back to it as quick as you can.

-Don't let the shoulders travel up towards the ears and create tension in the neck.

-Keep hips level.

-To help with balance, keep your eyes focused on a point on the floor that does not move.

*BURPEES:

1. Stand with your legs wider than your body.
2. Bend the knees, and bring your hands to the floor directly under the shoulders.
3. Step back with the right leg to bring it directly behind the right hip. Repeat with the left leg. You will end up in a plank formation.
   Progression: Hop both legs out simultaneously into plank position and add a push up.
4. Step right leg up and then back to its starting position. Repeat with the left leg to end in a tuck position.
   Progression: Hop both legs back in at the same time.
5. Stand up.

   Repeat as many times as you can without losing proper form.

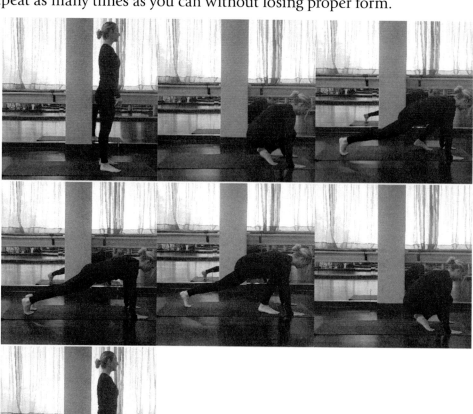

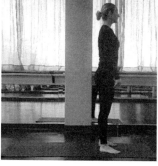

Burpee Notes:

-This can be a higher intensity exercise. If your body does not like this movement for whatever reason, please replace the exercise with a previous one from earlier in the week.

-Keep track of the number of repetitions you complete. The number of reps completed will be your "Mile Marker."

-Go at your comfortable pace. Remember, you want to push yourself-not hurt yourself.

Feeling stronger yet? Keep it up! Don't forget about your cool down on Page xix.

Week Three – Day Three

Ephesians 5:29-30

> *"After all, no one hated their own body, but they feed and care for their own body, just as Christ does the church for we are members of his body."*

Although this passage is meant as a teaching for how a man is to love his wife, I think it can speak a bold message to us in this program as well. Think about God's love for His church; His perfect, unconditional, never-failing love. Wouldn't it be nice to have that same love for ourselves? When human nature takes over, we can stare in the mirror and list all the physical qualities we would like to change. Some traits are the effects of poor daily habits and we can take measures to manage those. Other traits are God-given and should not be insulted.

Often, I overhear my clients complaining to each other about how they hate certain parts of their bodies. I want to cringe when I hear this. Hate is such a strong word and should be removed from our vocabulary when we talk about ourselves. Just as God's frustrations and disappointments with us never lead to hate, our feelings about ourselves shouldn't either. Respect yourself enough as God's creation to take "hate" out of your self-dialogue. We do ourselves no favors by casting out insults.

As Christians, we are members of Christ's body, so let's follow his example in how He cares for it. From the beginning, God has fed and nurtured the church. He tends to its needs. He supports and strengthens it. He always has and always will. What a powerful example! We must feed and care for our bodies; listening to and supporting its needs as well as honoring its limitations. Limitations don't equate to weakness; rather, it takes a strong and gracious person to take a step back when their pride tells them to step forward.

You are not perfect, but Jesus loves you anyway because you are a member of his body. Whatever flaws you have, seek to love them the same way. Read the passage from Ephesians again. Today, take strides to care for your body as Christ does the church- unconditionally.

DAY THREE FITNESS ROUTINES

Warm up is on Page xv for your reference.

*PUSH-UPS:

1. On the floor, place your hands a little wider than your shoulders. Bring your knees back past your hips, not under them. Engage abdominals to support the spine.
   Progression: Attempt push-ups with your knees lifted off of the floor.
   Modification: Push-ups can be done at an angle on a bathroom or kitchen countertop.
2. Slowly bend the elbow to lower the chest towards the floor. Take 3 counts to lower and then lift in 1 count to return to starting position. Three counts down, 1 count up. Repeat 5-10 times.
3. Repeat the movement taking single counts down and up. Repeat as many times as you are able while keeping proper form. *Keep track of the number of repetitions you complete for your "Mile Marker."

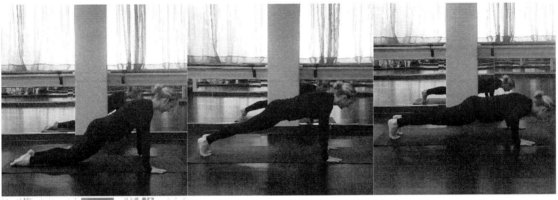

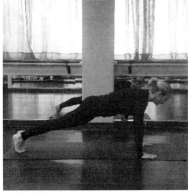

Push-up Notes:

-*Be cautious not to drop your head towards the floor. Remember, your head is an extension of the neck which is an extension of the spine.*

-*Move in your pain-free range of motion. Whatever your joints allow you to accomplish.*

-*Pictures are in the progression form.*

KNEELING SERIES:

1. Begin on your knees. Place your right hand on the floor directly under the shoulder. Extend the left leg to the side. Engage the core and lift bottom ribcage. Keep your head and neck extended.
    Modification: If your knees don't allow for the kneeling position, this series can be done lying on your side with your hips and shoulders stacked.
2. Lift the left leg to your highest comfortable position.
3. Slowly lower the leg diagonally to the front to tap the toe on the floor. *Modification: Don't lower all the way to the floor if your hips come unstacked.*
4. Lift the leg back to your highest point in line with your body.
5. Slowly lower the leg diagonally to the back to tap the floor with your foot. *Modification: If you feel your hips opening too much and becoming unstacked, don't lower all the way to the floor.*
6. Return the leg back to your highest point in line with your body. Repeat 5-10 times.
7. Rest if needed and reset in position with your leg in line with your hip. Reach the leg long to the left.
    Modification: Bend at the knee to shorten the lever to ease the intensity.
8. Moving in a circular motion from your hip (not your knee) trace a soccer ball sized circle with your big toe. Repeat 5-10 times.
9. Reverse the circular motion and complete 5-10 rotations.
10. Rest and repeat on the other side.

    Rest if needed and repeat series 1-2 more times.

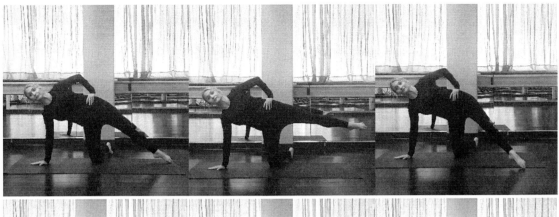

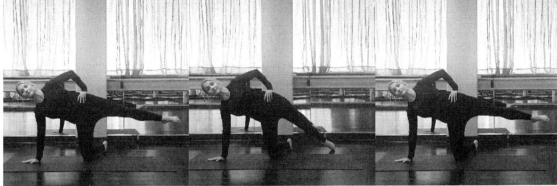

Kneeling Series Notes:

-Picture a large triangle to your sides and trace it with your big toe.

-As always, move in your pain-free range of motion.

-As your body fatigues, the motion will start to move from the hip and into the knee. Stay strong and keep the movement in the hip joints.

-Keep the supporting knee under the hip.

-Keep movement out of torso. This is only from the waist down.

STARFISH CRUNCHES:

1. Start by lying on your back with arms over head in a "V" shape, palms facing the ceiling. Open legs to your widest comfortable width.
2. Engage your abdominals. Take 4 counts to lift your head, right arm, and right shoulder blade from the floor at the same time lifting the left leg. Twisting in the torso, tap your leg with your fingertips.

Modification: Leave the head and shoulder blades on the floor. You may also bend the arms and legs to shorten the lever, easing the intensity if needed.

3. Take 4 counts to lower the upper body and lower body to the floor simultaneously.
4. Repeat using the left upper body and right leg. Repeat 4-6 times.
5. Repeat another 4-6 times using 2 counts for each movement.
    Modification: Stay with the slower 4 count pace.

Repeat series 2-3 times.

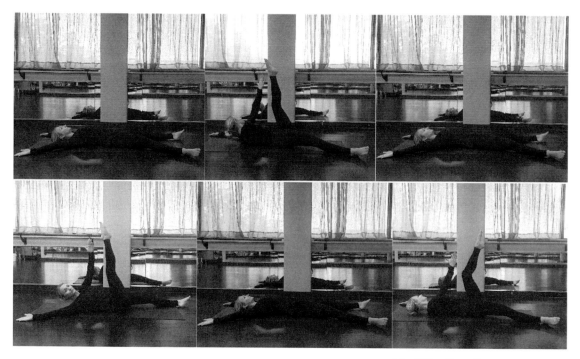

Modification Form

Starfish Crunch Notes:

-*Embrace the modifications to ease any tension in the neck, shoulders, or hips.*

-*Make sure the movements from the legs and arms are at the same time. As you get tired, they may start to move separately.*

CALF RAISES:

1. If needed, stand close to something that can help you balance, a chair for example. With your heels together and toes apart, stretch the spine upwards and engage your abdominals in a baring down motion.
2. Lift the heels off of the floor engaging your calf muscles. Feel the weight dispersed evenly amongst the balls of your feet and all ten toes.
3. Slowly, with control, lower the heels to the floor. Resist the temptation to rock back to your heels. Repeat 8 times.
4. Lift your heels and then only lower half-way down to the floor. Repeat 8 times.
5. Lift your heels and pulse just an inch or so in a bouncing motion. Continue for a count of 16.

   Repeat series 2-3 times.

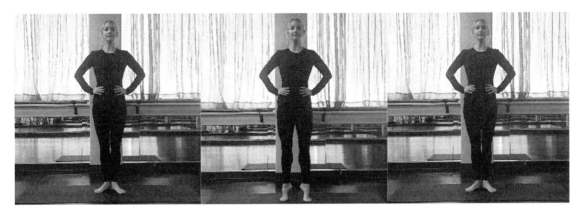

Calf Raise Notes:

-Feel free to take a break when needed and roll the ankle. This exercise will strengthen both the muscle and joint. Honor your body when it needs a break!

-This can also be done in a parallel position with the toes in front of the heels.

You are half-way through the week. Way to go! Cool down is next.

Week Three – Day Four

Proverbs 16:24

> *"Gracious words are a honeycomb, sweet to the soul and healing to the bones."*

There is no coincidence in the comparison of gracious words and honeycomb in this passage. As we grow wiser with age, we learn that there is power in our words. We can make someone's day or ruin it by the words that come out of our mouths. The same goes for us in the way we think about ourselves. In renewing your mind to think kind thoughts about yourself, true healing is taking place. Today's passage tells us that gracious words are like honeycomb; let's take a quick and practical look into what medical professionals are currently saying about honey:

- It is an anti-microbial.
- It is an anti-inflammatory.
- It assists in insulin production.
- It is an anti-fungal.
- It can be used to treat certain eye conditions.
- It is a cough suppressant.
- It has been found to help in cancer prevention.
- It is an anti-viral.
- It can help prevent cardiovascular disease.
- It can be used to help oral hygiene.

The benefits are truly impressive. If kind, gracious words are healing like honey, we need to start pouring them out wherever we go! And not just to others but also to ourselves. As we learn to honor God with our bodies, we start to find a whole new appreciation for our vessels. Our physical attributes, our abilities, even our disabilities of all kinds become more valued as we view our bodies as a form of worship. As you go about your day, be mindful to have a honey-filled impact in your community. Take that honeycomb of kindness and drizzle that sweet stuff over yourself as well. You are important. Your health is important and it is worth all the effort you are putting into it.

Before you move to today's exercises, read the verse one more time. Kind words are healing. Satan wants us beaten and broken down. Make the effort to uplift yourself and others in your life.

DAY FOUR FITNESS ROUTINE

Please refer to Page xv for your warm up.

LUNGES:

1. Standing with your head over your shoulders, your shoulders over your hips, and your hips over your ankles, place your hands on your hips.
2. Engage the abdominal muscles by hugging them around your spine- feeling it in the front, back and sides.
3. Place an imaginary string on top of your head and allow it to pull you taller towards the ceiling.
4. Step back with the right leg, placing the ball of your foot on the floor (heel is lifted).
   Modification: For help with balance, place a chair to the side of you and hold a lightly.
   Progression: Lift front heel as well.
5. Bending both knees, bring the right knee closer towards the floor.
6. Hold this lunge position.
   Progression: Attempt to pulse a little lower 5-10 times.
7. Step together.
8. Repeat on the left side. Repeat 10-15 times.

Rest if needed and repeat the series 2-3 times.

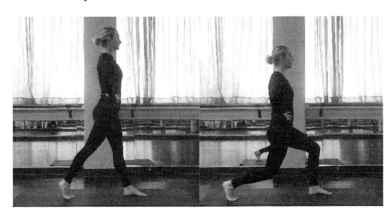

Lunge Notes:

-Be cautious not to hinge forward from the waste. Keep shoulders over hips throughout the series.

-As you step back, allow the front leg to shift back at the hip as well. When you bend into your lunges, look down and make sure your front knee in aligned with your ankle.

-Work in your pain-free range of motion. If your knees don't bend much, don't force it!

*TRICEP PUSH-UPS:

1. Starting on all fours, place your hands directly under the shoulders with the fingers pointing forward. Bring your knees back past your hips. Engage the core so the spine does not dip towards the floor. Your neck is long.
   Progression: Lift the knees from the floor into a full push-up position.
2. Taking 3 counts, bend at the elbows allowing the arms to brush the sides of your body as your torso lowers towards the floor.
3. Take a single count to extend the arms to return to starting position. Repeat 4-6 times.
4. Reverse the counts. Take 1 count to lower the body and 3 counts to extend at the elbow to raise the body. Repeat 4-6 times.
5. Continue the same motion, taking 1 count down and 1 count to come up. Repeat as many times as you can while keeping proper form.

   Repeat series 1-3 times.

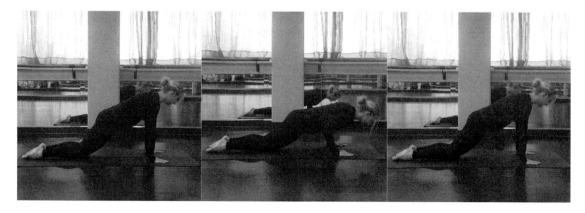

Tricep Push-up Notes:

-*Due to the difficulty level of this exercise, the number of repetitions you are able to complete is your "Mile Marker."*

-*Do not drop your head towards the floor.*

-*Keep the abdominals engaged to support the spine.*

-*Tell yourself to squeeze your ribs with your elbows. This will help you keep the arms close to the body.*

-*Allow the elbows to bend in such a way that they are "pointing" in the direction of your toes.*

ROLLING LIKE A BALL: (THIS ONE IS FUN!)

1. Sit on the floor. Look behind you and make sure there is nothing in your way. We will be rolling back and I don't want you to hit anything.
2. Sit up nice and tall, your knees towards your chest, feet flat on the floor, and your hands on top of your shins.
3. Lift your heels from the floor and lower your chin to your chest to round out your spine. Lean back slightly and lift your toes few inches. You are now in your ball position.
   Modification: Holding this pose takes a lot of deep core strength. If you need to, feel free to hold this position instead of adding the movement that will follow.
4. Keep your chin tucked and knees as close as you can to your chest. Roll back onto your shoulder blades.
5. Roll up into the starting position. Hold for 3 seconds then begin to roll back again. Repeat 5-10 times.
6. Hold at the top of your last roll. Lift the chin from the chest to straighten the spine. Extend your legs and take your palms around the back of your calves. Hold this position for 10-20 seconds.
   Progression: Open your legs to a "V" position. For an extra challenge, attempt your rolling action in this "V" shape.

Rest if needed and repeat the series 2-3 times.

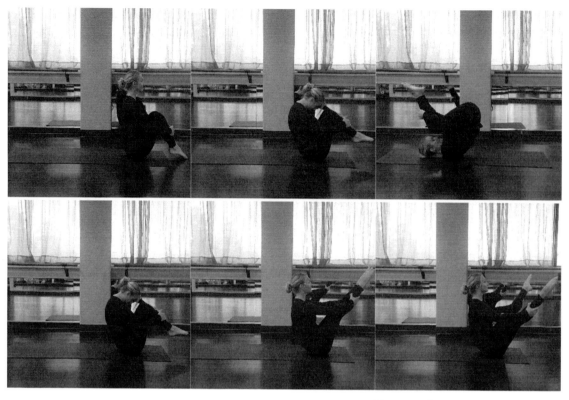

Progression

Rolling Like A Ball Notes:

-Be cautious not to roll back onto your neck. Keep the pressure in your shoulder blades as you roll back onto the floor.

-As you roll up, the legs might want to come away from your body to assist your torso. Keep them pulled in tight.

-Make sure you hold at the top of the roll before you go back for your next one. Otherwise, you're just rocking with gravity and momentum doing all the work.

-You may shift as you roll. Be aware of your surroundings so you don't hit your head on anything.

REVERSE CRUNCHES:

1. Lay on your back with your legs lifted towards the ceiling and keep your knees soft. Cross your legs at the ankles and place your hands under your tailbone.

2. Lift your tailbone from the floor and allow it to quickly return down. Do not swing the legs back and forth. It is a quick up and down motion. Repeat 10-15 times.

3. Repeat the movement at a slower pace- 1 count to lift the hips up and 1 count to lower them to the floor. Repeat 5-10 times.

Repeat series 2-4 times.

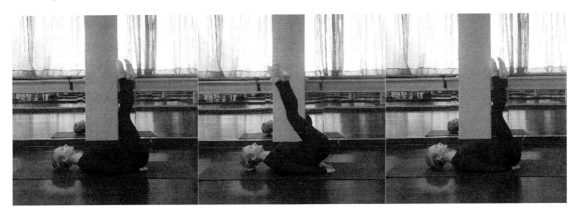

Reverse Crunch Notes:

-Stay light in the arms. Do not press down too hard into the floor. This may cause tension in the neck and shoulders.

-Don't worry about controlling the hips down on the first set. Allow the hips to drop down quickly. The control comes into play when you slow it down on the second round. Feel the spine peel up off of the floor as you lift the hips. Then you use your lower abdominals to control the hips down, lowering one vertebra at a time.

-Watch the angles of your hip and knee joints. Make sure they aren't expanding as you lift your hips. If they are, that simply means you are trying to use momentum from your legs to assist the lift. Allow all the effort to come from your abdominals.

-If your hips start to feel tight, bend your knees more to shorten the lever.

Good work today. Learn to love the burn! Now go reward your body with your cool down.

Week Three – Day Five

Lamentations 3:22-23

> *"Because of the Lord's great love we are not consumed, for his compassions never fail. They are new every morning; great is your faithfulness."*

Our Lord is a merciful Lord and His gracious mercies are new to us every day. When I first started the practice of viewing my body as a vessel of worship, I tried to bestow new mercies onto myself to follow God's example. When I woke up, I would tell myself, "Okay Kara, you might have slipped up a few times yesterday but today is a new day. You've got this!" Over time, I noticed I had to give myself grace more than just in the morning. Sometimes I would have to give myself a little pep talk a couple of times a day, sometimes hourly, sometimes minute-by-minute. I found it was crucial to the success of the program to realize that I'm not perfect at this yet; but I was trying. Being years into this practice, I still have to let the grace flow from time to time.

As you go about your days, seek opportunities to bestow grace and mercy to yourself. If you give in to temptation, don't be cruel to yourself. Instead, simply acknowledge the lapse and tell yourself to try harder next time- because, most likely, there will be a next time. We won't get it right all the time; we are human after all. We are not perfect but that is ok because we serve a God that is!

Take a moment to read today's verse again. Because God loves you so much, His mercies will never leave you. Every morning when you get out of bed, you are new and flawless in His eyes. It is as if we have a reset button. Learn to give yourself that same grace. It is okay to hit your reset button.

DAY FIVE FITNESS ROUTINE - WEIGHTED SERIES

Please refer to Page xv for your warm up.

Weights are not required for these series but are recommended to fully maximize your efforts. If you have two sets of weights, start with the heavier then switch to the lighter set as you need.

OVERHEAD BICEP CURL SERIES:

1. Standing, bend your arms to bring your elbows behind the back, palms facing up. Relax the shoulders down the spine and engage the core.
2. Keeping the bend in your arms, take 2 counts to lift the arms up diagonally. The arms are not directly over the head. If you look up without lifting your chin, you should be able to see your weights.
3. Take 2 counts to lower the arms down to starting position. Repeat 4-8 times and stop your arms half-way down on your last repetition.
4. Take 1 count to lift your arms diagonally overhead.
5. Take 1 count to lower your arms half-way down. Repeat 6-10 times.
6. Return the arms to starting position with the elbows behind the back.
7. Quickly extend the arms (keeping them below shoulder height) and return the elbows back behind the body. Repeat 10-15 times.

Repeat the series 2-3 times.

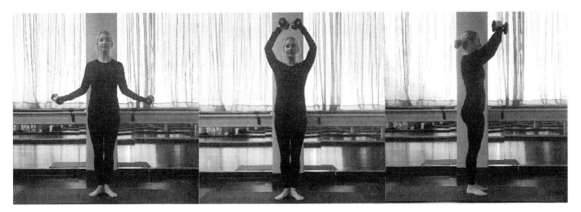

Side View

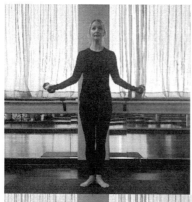

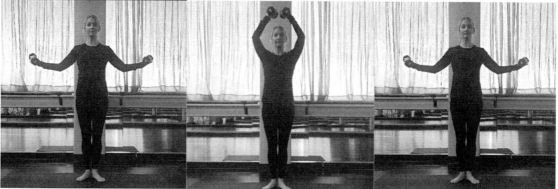

Overhead Bicep Curl Notes:

-As you lift overhead, keep the abdominals tight so the ribcage doesn't move away from the spine.

-Move in your pain-free range of motion.

-Keep the shoulders down the spine so tension doesn't build in the neck area.

DEADLIFTS:

1. Stand with your legs under the hips and toes forward. Soften your knees and hinge the upper body to a flat back position. Extend your arms towards the floor directly under the shoulders. Keep neck extended.
   Modification: If flat back isn't an option for you, hinge to your lowest comfortable position.
2. At your own pace, lift the torso and straighten the legs simultaneously. Engage the glutes.
3. Again, at your own pace, return to starting hinged position. Repeat 5-10 times.
4. Staying in your hinged position, lift the torso an inch then lower an inch. Repeat the pulse 5-10 times.

   Repeat series 2-3 times.

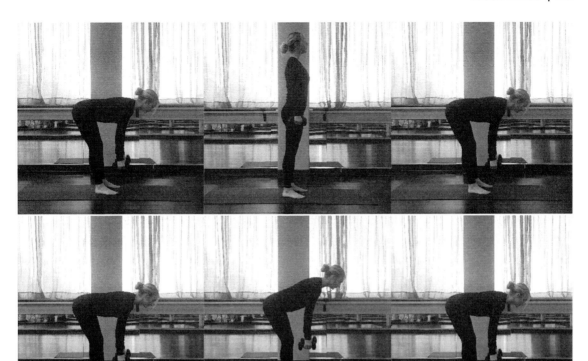

Deadlift Notes:

-Keep the shoulders rolled back and pressed down the spine.

-Don't drop the head.

-Abdominals need to stay tight to support the hinged spine.

TRICEP "V'S":

1. Stand with your arms extended towards the ceiling, palms facing front. Lower the chin towards the chest. Open the arms to a "V" position.
   Modification: Lower arms towards the floor and open in a "V" position with palms facing behind.
2. Bend at the elbows to lower the weights behind the head.
   Modification: Bend at the elbows to bring the weights towards the under arms.
3. Extend the arms and reach back out to the "V" position. Repeat 5-10 times.

   Rest if needed and repeat the series 2-3 times.

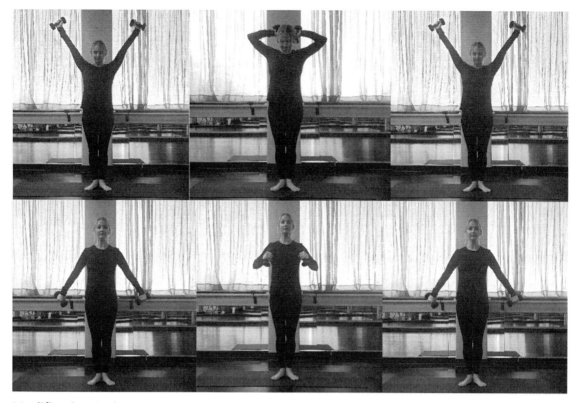

Modification Series

Tricep "V" Notes:

-As you extend the arms overhead, keep the ribcage pulled in towards the spine.

-Fully extend to properly engage the muscles in the back of the arm.

-Make sure you control the weights as they travel down. Don't let gravity pull them down quickly.

CHEST PRESS & SHOULDER RAISES:

1. Stand with the ends of your weights pressing against each other. Soften you elbows. Roll the shoulders back and press them low down the back.
2. Take 2 counts to lift the arms front to shoulder height (or to your highest comfortable point).
3. Take 2 counts to lower the arms back to starting position. Repeat 4-8 times and hold at the top of your last repetition.
4. Take 1 count to lower the arms half-way down.

5. Take 1 count to lift back to shoulder height. Repeat 4-8 times.
6. Keeping arms at your highest comfortable point, lower the arms an inch then lift an inch. Repeat 4-8 times.

Repeat series 2-3 times.

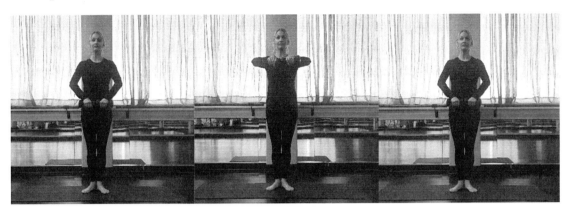

Chest Press & Shoulder Raise Notes:

-Keep the ends of your weights pressed together throughout the series to engage the chest muscles.

-Move in your pain-free range of motion.

-Don't let the shoulders travel up and create tension in the neck area.

Your body, heart, mind, and soul are transforming. Keep it up!

Week Three – Day Six

Isaiah 43:18-19

> *"Forget the former things: do not dwell in the past. See, I am doing a new thing! Now it springs up; do you not perceive it? I am making a way in the wilderness and streams in the wasteland."*

What a power-packed message! There are three main points to be taken away from these verses.

1) God wants us to focus on the future. If you are like me, you have been on and off the "healthy" band wagon. Satan wants to use those past failures to discourage any future advances in your healthy lifestyle, especially if you're on fire for the Lord. Don't allow Satan to distract and discourage you with your past. Keep your eyes on the prize- a healthier, happier you that is capable of serving God better and longer.

2) God is currently active in your life; "See, I am doing a new thing! Now it springs up...". God is at work in your life today and every day. Join Him in creating a better life for you and your community. Allow Him to use you in His great and undeniably mighty plans. The Lord put *A Body of Worship* in my heart and in your hands for a reason. Let's not waste it.

3) God makes a way when all seems hopeless. In the reality of the broken world, our lives are like the overgrown trees and shrubbery of the wilderness from the passage- impossible to trek through on our own. As we progress through this program, we may, at times, feel that we are in that jungle not knowing which way to go or where to turn; feeling vulnerable to an attack at any time. Scripture says that God is making a path through the challenges. Lean on Him and follow His way. We are not on this journey alone. Next week, we will look deeper into this realization that God is with us every step of the way.

Take a moment to read the verse again. Can you picture it? The clear path in the overgrown jungle? The beautiful stream in the desert? God is working in your life. Open your eyes and watch His greatness unfold.

DAY SIX FITNESS ROUTINE

Refer to Page xv for your warm up.

SWAN PUSH UP:

1. Lying on your stomach, place your hands on the floor outside of your shoulders. With a natural turnout in your hips, extend your legs to reach behind you. Reach the ears away from the tops of the shoulders and keep your eyes focused towards the floor.
2. Take 2 counts and simultaneously use your arms to press up and the lower back to lift the chest from the floor. Keep your elbows close to your body.
   Progression: Lift the legs from the floor at the same time as the upper body.
3. Take 2 counts to lower back to starting position with control. Repeat 5-10 times.
4. Take 1 count to lift the upper body.
5. Take 1 count to lower down. Repeat 8-12 times.

   Repeat series 2-3 times.

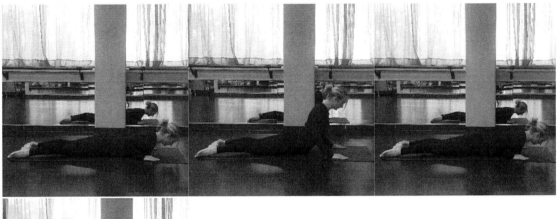

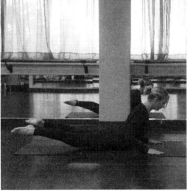

Progression Form

Swan Push Up Notes:

-There is no need to fully extend the arms. Only press up to a point that is comfortable to your low back.

- Imagine a flashlight on the tip of your nose. The light should be shining to the floor during this entire exercise which will eliminate movement in the neck. All movement should be in the arms and low back. If you're lifting your legs as well, the glutes will be activated.

SIDE PLANK:

1. Lay on your right side with your elbow on the floor under the shoulder. Palm on the floor. Left hand on your left hip. Bend your bottom leg to a comfortable position. Top leg extended straight.
   Progression: Place your hand under your shoulder with your right arm straight. For further intensity, you may also keep both legs extended with top foot staggered on the floor in front of bottom foot.
2. Using your abdominals, take 2 counts to lift your hips from the floor. Extend your left arm up and reach overhead. Look up towards your fingers.
3. Lower the hips back towards the floor in 2 counts. Hand returns to hip. Repeat 8-10 times.
4. Repeat on the other side. Repeat 8-10 times.

   Repeat series 2-3 times.

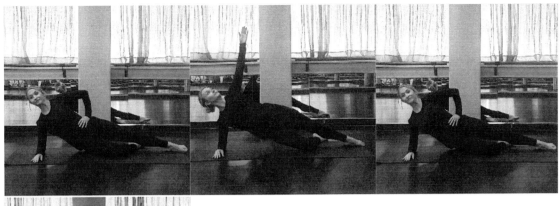

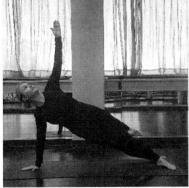

Progression Form

Side Plank Notes:

-Don't allow the head to drop towards the shoulder. You want to keep your neck extended to prevent tension.

-Engage the bottom oblique abdominals to properly lift the hips and ribcage.

PILLOW PASSES:

1. Grab a small pillow (or a comparable object) and lie on your back. Extend legs in front and arms overhead behind you with pillow in hands.
2. Slowly lift both legs at the same time towards the ceiling. While you are lifting your legs, raise the arms, head, and shoulder blades from the floor. Pass the pillow from the hands to in between the knees.
   Modification: Keep the head and shoulder blades on the floor and just move the arms and legs. You may also bend the legs to shorten the lever easing the intensity, if needed.

3. Slowly and simultaneously lower back down to the floor to starting position. Allow the spine to arch naturally from the floor and fully relax the body before the next repetition.
4. Repeat and pass the pillow from the legs to the hands.
5. Repeat the Pillow Pass 15-30 times.

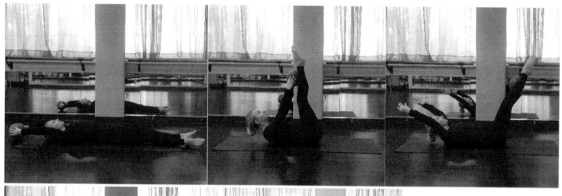

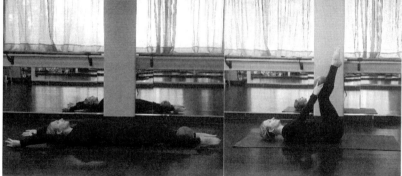

Modification Form

Pillow Pass Notes:

-If your hips begin to feel tight, bend at the knees and do not lower the legs all the way to the floor.

-Keep the chin lifted away from the chest.

-With this exercise, the slower the movement, the more effective it will be. Slower is better!

JAZZ HAND SQUATS:

1. Stand with your legs wider than your hips. Bring your hands into prayer position in front of the chest.
2. Hinge forward from the waist as you bend your knees slightly to a half-squat position. Hold.
3. Open your hands and move them so the palms face away from your body. Bend the knees a little lower and attempt to bring your elbows to tap the tops of your thighs. *Modification: Refrain from lowering too far down if you have limited range of motion.*
4. Fully extend into starting position with hands returning to prayer.

   Repeat 10-30 times.

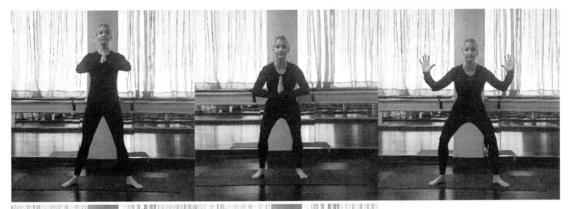

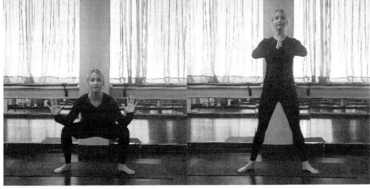

Week Three is complete. Great job staying dedicated!

Don't forget to cool down.

WEEK FOUR

A Body of Worship is never alone.

Week Four – Day One

Psalm 16:8

> *"I keep my eyes always on the Lord. With him at my right hand, I will not be shaken."*

What a powerful passage with three major points:

1. We must keep our focus on the Lord.
2. He is next to us through it all.
3. And when God is with us, we will not be defeated.

My two-year-old enjoys playing in her room by herself from time to time. I use these moments to do the dishes, fold laundry, or whatever task I've been trying to complete all day. And, although I'm not in there playing with her, I'm watching her either on the room monitor or stealthily peeking in on her. I know she is safe and content. But when something happens and she calls out to me, I run quickly to assess the situation. Most likely, she just wants to show me a toy or to know I'm still around, but I run with urgency towards her every time. When my daughter is not distracted and her focus is on me, I'm right by her side and she knows she is safe. The same is true for us and our Heavenly Father.

When our focus is where it should be, we are unstoppable because the Lord will not forsake us. During the past three weeks, we have learned what it means to have *A Body of Worship*; we are sacrificial, self-disciplined, self-controlled, renewed and full of grace. Today, we adopt a new discipline- focus. We focus our efforts towards a healthier life for God. The Lord put us on this earth for a reason, and we must be diligent and stay focused to be healthy enough to finish our tasks.

Before heading into your fitness routine for today, re-read the Bible verse. Where is your focus? Keep your eyes on the Lord through it all and you will come out on top.

DAY ONE FITNESS ROUTINE

If needed, refer to Page xv for your warm up.

WALK THE PLANK:

1. Start by standing in a place with plenty of room in front of you. legs hip distance apart and arms down by your sides.
2. As you inhale, circle your arms overhead and stretch towards the ceiling.
3. As you exhale, lower the arms in front and forward fold. Bring your hands as close to the floor as you can.
4. Bend your knees to lower into a tuck position.
   Modification: If your knees do not allow for a full tuck, just bend to a position that is comfortable for you.
5. With your hands on the floor, walk out to a plank position.
   Modification: Lower to the knees first then walk out to a knee plank position.
6. Hold plank for 5-10 seconds. *Progression: Add 3-6 push-ups.*
7. Bend your knees and walk the hands back towards the feet to return to your tuck.
8. Slowly roll up one vertebra at a time, allowing the head to be the last thing to lift.

   Repeat series 5-15 times.

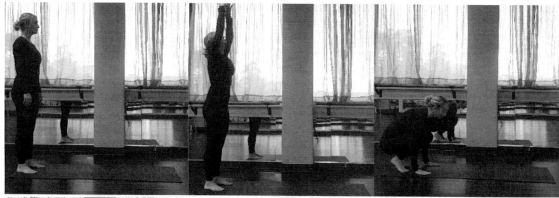

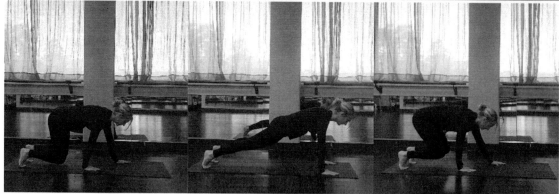

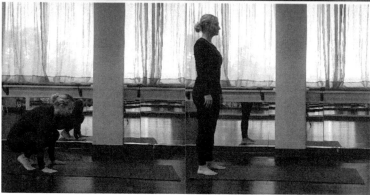

Walk the Plank Notes:

-Keep a slow pace unless you feel comfortable with the movement and you would like to add a cardio aspect to this exercise. If so, you may increase your speed.

-As you are walking in and out of your tuck position, make sure the hips are not swaying side to side too much. I tell my clients to make sure they are not "wagging their tails." Keep abdominals engaged to manage this.

CALF RAISES:

1. If needed, stand close to something that can help you balance, a chair for example. With your heels together and toes apart, stretch the spine upwards and engage your abdominals in a baring down motion.
2. Lift the heels off of the floor engaging your calf muscles. Feel the weight dispersed evenly amongst the balls of your feet and all ten toes.
3. Slowly, with control, lower the heels to the floor. Resist the temptation to rock back to your heels. Repeat 8 times.
4. Lift your heels and then only lower half-way down to the floor. Repeat 8 times.
5. Lift your heels and pulse just an inch or so in a bouncing motion. Continue for a count of 16.

Repeat series 2-3 times.

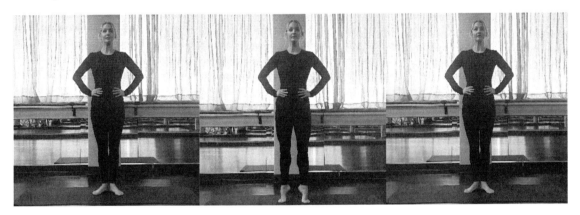

Calf Raise Notes:

-Feel free to take a break when needed and roll the ankle. This exercise will strengthen both the muscles and joints. Honor your body when it needs a break!

-This can also be done in a parallel position with the toes in front of the heels.

STANDING SIDE CRUNCHES:

1. Stand with your legs wide apart and turned out from the hips. Bend the knees to your lowest comfortable position. Roll the hips up towards the ribcage to neutralize your spine and then engage your abdominals in a baring down motion. Bring your hands behind your head with your elbows opened to the sides.

Progression: Slightly lean back to further engage abdominals.
Modification: Slightly lean forward to ease abdominal engagement.

2. At your own pace, crunch laterally to the right. Feel the side abdominals (the obliques) contract.
3. Using the left side obliques, lift the torso to return directly over hips.
4. Repeat on the right side 20-40 times.
5. Repeat the series crunching to the left 20-40 times.

   Rest and repeat the series 2-3 times.

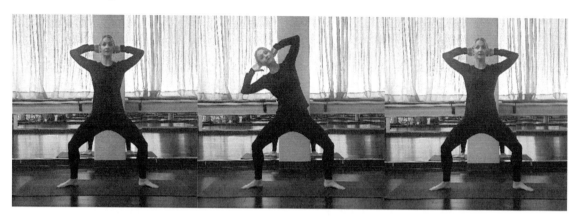

Standing Side Crunch Notes:

-*The goal of this exercise is to get the elbows as close as you can to your thighs without lowering your arms.*

-*Go at your own comfortable pace and range of motion.*

-*Stay low in your legs to engage the glutes and quadriceps.*

-*It is important to keep the abdominals tight to support the lateral flexion of the spine.*

BRIDGES:

1. Lay on your back and place your feet flat on the floor with your ankles under your knees. Legs will need to be a little wider than your body. Place your arms by your side.
   Modification: If your knees don't allow for that range of motion, bring your feet forward away from the body until you find a comfortable position.
   Progression: Lift the heels off of the floor and press the balls of your feet down. Lift arms towards ceiling.

2. Roll the hips up towards the ribcage until the spine is flat on the floor.
3. Engage your glute muscles and lift the hips towards the ceiling.
4. Take 2 counts to relax the glutes and return to starting position by rolling down the spine one vertebra at a time.
5. Take 2 counts to engage the glutes and roll through the spine to return the hips up. Repeat 4-8 times.
6. Continue the same motion, taking 1 count to lower and 1 count to lift the hips. Repeat 8-12 times. Hold at the top of your last lift.
7. Tighten the glutes slightly harder to lift the hips about an inch. Then slightly release the contraction to lower them about an inch. Continue the small pulses 10-14 times.

Repeat series 2-3 times.

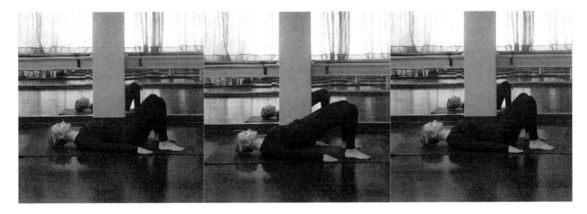

Bridge Notes:

-Create opposition by pressing feet firmly into the floor. This will engage the back of the thighs (your hamstrings).

-You should never feel pressure in your neck. If you do, lower the seat down until you only feel the weight in your upper back.

- Keep your glutes engaged while at the top of your bridge to maximize the benefits of this exercise; only relax the muscles when you return to the floor.

Fantastic work! Keep up the self-discipline as you go about your day today.

Cool Down is on Page xix for your reference.

Week Four – Day Two

Isaiah 40:29-31

> *"He gives strength to the weary and increases the power of the weak. Even youths grow tired and weary, and young men stumble and fall; but those who hope in the Lord will renew their strength. They will soar on wings like eagles; they will run and not grow weary, they will walk and not be faint."*

It is inevitable; you will stumble and make mistakes as you strive to become a stronger and healthier individual. Give yourself grace during these times and put your hope and trust in the Lord because when you do so, you will succeed. Lean on God when you grow weary and allow Him to strengthen you. Put in the effort and the discipline, but most importantly put God in the middle of it all and watch Him work in you. If you are doing this program with a friend or family member, you know how encouraging it is to have a support system. If you're doing this alone, there may be times when you feel overwhelmed. Know that whether you have five people or none along with you on this journey, you are never alone. God is in your corner and so proud of the work you are putting in for your health and His kingdom.

Read the verse above one more time. Picture yourself with the endurance God wants to give you- that alone is re-energizing. When you feel weak, remember why you started. Find your strength in the Lord and you will soar!

DAY TWO FITNESS ROUTINE – WEIGHTED EXERCISES

-Start with heavier weights and feel free to move to a lighter weight at any point. Weights are not required but recommended to maximize your results.

Please refer to Page xv for your warm up.

SIDE BICEP CURLS:

1. Stand with your feet hip distance apart and core engaged. Bring your elbows to your ribcage with your palms facing up.
2. Extend your arms to the sides and lift your elbows to shoulder height.
   Modification: Lift your elbows only as high as comfortable if you have shoulder discomfort.
3. Flex at the elbow joint, bringing the hands towards the shoulders.
4. Extend the arms back out.
5. Lower the elbows back to the ribcage. Repeat 10-15 times.
6. Shortening your range of motion (not lifting as high), pulse the extension of the arms; quickly extending the arms and then quickly returning them to the ribcage. Repeat 10-15 times.

Repeat series 2-4 times.

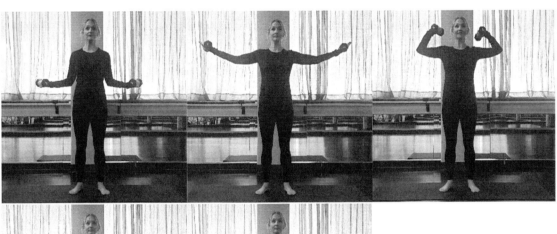

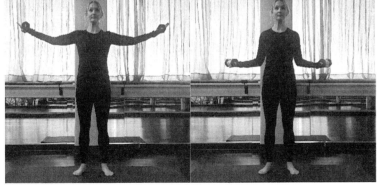

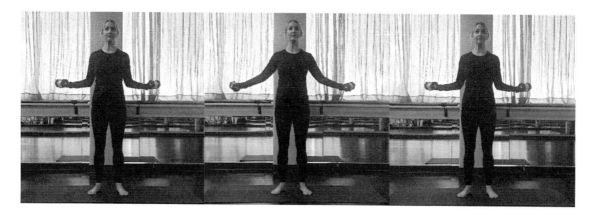

Side Bicep Curl Notes:

-When you lift and extend the arms, keep your abdominals tight and your ribcage pulled in towards the spine.

-Work in your pain-free range of motion.

-Stay strong in the wrists. Don't allow the weight to pull the knuckles down.

WEIGHTED FLIES:

1. Stand with your feet hip distance apart, bend knees, and hinge forward from the hips. Engage abdominals to support your spine. Depress shoulders down the back. Allow your eyes to focus on the floor a few feet in front of you to keep the neck long. With your weights in hand, hug an imaginary beach ball in front of your chest.
2. Take 2 counts to open the arms to the sides as if the beach ball is getting bigger. Feel the shoulder blades moving towards the spine.
3. Take 2 counts to lower the arms to starting position. Repeat 8 times.
4. Repeat the same movement taking single counts to lift and lower the arms. Repeat 8 times.
5. Lift arms to your highest comfortable position and pulse the arms half-way down. Repeat 16 times.

   Repeat series 1-3 times.

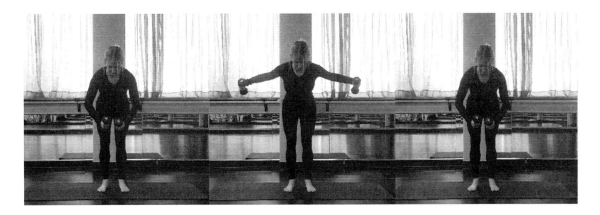

Weighted Fly Notes:

-Be cautious not to allow the abdominals to disengage. This will cause the spine to drop and create tension in the low back.

-While lowering the shoulder blades down the spine, reach the ears away from the shoulders to keep the neck long.

-Move in your pain-free range of motion.

-Keep the body's weight in your heels. You should be able to wiggle your toes.

TRICEP LIFTS:

1. Return to your hinge position. Stand with your ankles directly under your hips. Bend your knees and hinge forward from the hips. Slightly tilt the pelvis forward and engage the abdominals. Roll the shoulders back/around/and down; chest is proud. Reach the shoulders low down the spine. The neck is long.
2. Extend the arms towards the floor directly under the shoulders, palms facing each other.
3. Take 2 counts to lift the arms behind to your highest comfortable point.
4. Take 2 counts to lower the arms to starting position. Repeat 5-10 times.
5. Take 2 counts to lift just the right arm behind you.
6. Take 2 counts to return the right arm down. Repeat 5-10 times.
7. Repeat on the left side 5-10 times.

   Repeat series 2-3 times.

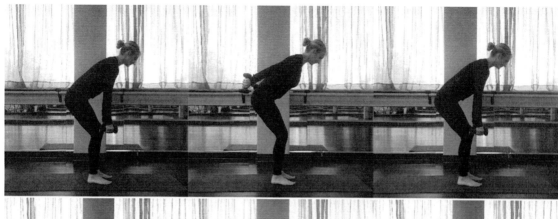

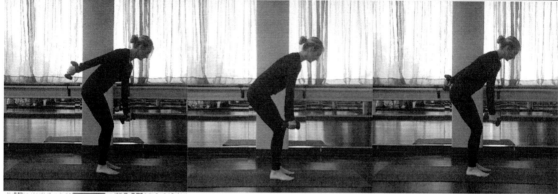

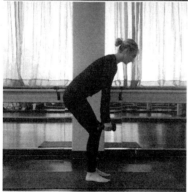

Tricep Lift Notes:

-*Work in your pain-free range of motion.*

-*If you need to go slower, please do so.*

-*If tension builds up in the neck, check your position. Are your shoulders slowly creeping up? Is your head dropping?*

-*Keep your core engaged to support the hinged spine.*

-*Keep the body weight in the back of the feet. Try wiggling your toes to check for this.*

-*Be cautious not to allow the arms to swing past the shoulders as you lower them.*

SHOULDER LIFTS WITH TORSO TWISTS:

1. Stand with your legs hip distant apart, arms down in front of your body and the palms towards the thighs.
2. Lift the arms straight up in front to shoulder height.
   Modification: Bend the arms to shorten the lever. If shoulder height is too high, lower to a comfortable position.
3. Engage the core and twist the whole upper body towards the right. Move at your comfortable pace and range of motion.
4. Twist back to the front.
5. Slowly lower the arms to starting position.
6. Lift the arms in front.
7. Engage the core and twist the upper body towards the left.
8. Twist back to the front.
9. Slowly lower the arms back down.

   Repeat each side 10-15 times.

   Rest then repeat the series 2-4 more times.

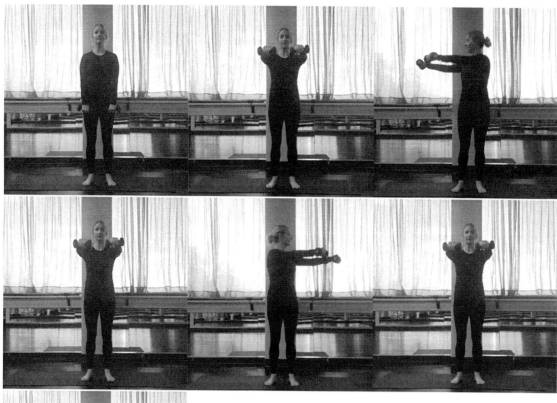

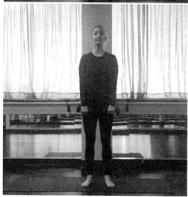

Shoulder Lift with Torso Twist Notes:

-Keep the shoulders depressed down the spine to minimize tension forming.

-Keep the core engaged to support the twisting motion of the spine.

You rocked it today! Treat your body to a cool down.

Week Four – Day Three

2 Thessalonians 3:3

> *"But the Lord is faithful, and he will strengthen you and protect you from the evil one."*

The evil one wants you weak. He wants you to stumble, fall, and not get up. The stronger you are spiritually, physically, and emotionally, the weaker the evil one becomes. The devil is lurking around the corner and putting obstacles in your way. Good thing for you, you are stronger than ever and you can jump right over those obstacles he puts in front of you. You are honoring your body with healthy eating, exercise, and putting God in the middle of it all!

Why does Satan want us to fail? For so many reasons, but I truly believe his main purpose is to separate us from God. Think about a time you have fallen short. A time when you thought you truly put it all in God's hands and still were unsuccessful. What happened next? The doubts and the questioning! "Why didn't God help me?"; "Why would God put this on my heart and not help to see it through?" The questions can go on and on. Sometimes success was not meant to happen at that moment; maybe your timing was not lined up with God's. Quite possibly you did begin your quest by putting it in God's hands, but ended up picking it back up by yourself without even noticing. Whatever the case may be, know that when your will lines up with God's, there is nothing Satan can do to stop you.

The Bible says the Lord is faithful to strengthen you in your weakest moments. Take hold of that promise and cherish it. The evil one is out there trying to derail you from your goals, but being aware of this fact gives you a major advantage. You can expect to be challenged and you can also expect to find strength in the Lord. With Him, there is nothing the devil can put in front of you that you cannot soar over.

Before moving on to today's exercise portion, take a moment to re-read the verse above. As you go about your day today, be aware that the evil one is waiting for a weak moment to distract and discourage you. Stand strong in your faith; know that Jesus will protect you from his schemes.

DAY THREE FITNESS ROUTINE

Please refer to Page xv if needed for your warm up.

*BURPEES:

1. Stand with your legs wider than your body.
2. Bend the knees, and bring your hands to the floor directly under the shoulders.
3. Step back with the right leg to bring it directly behind the right hip. Repeat with the left leg. You will end up in a plank formation.
    Progression: Hop both legs out simultaneously into plank position and add a push up.
4. Step right leg up and then back to its starting position. Repeat with the left leg to end in a tuck position.
    Progression: Hop both legs back in at the same time.
5. Stand up.

Repeat as many times as you can without losing proper form.

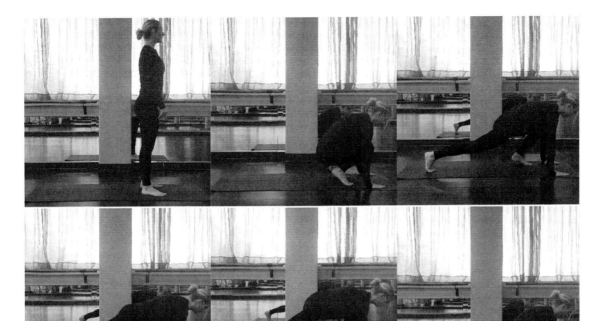

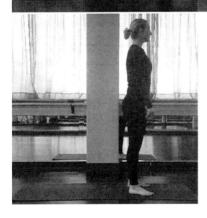

Burpee Notes:

-This can be a higher intensity exercise. If your body does not like this move for whatever reason, please replace this exercise with a previous one from earlier in the week.

-Keep track of the number of repetitions you complete. The number of reps completed will be your "Mile Marker."

-Go at your comfortable pace. Remember, you want to push yourself-not hurt yourself!

ROLL-UPS:

1. Lying on your back, bring your feet as close to your seat as you comfortably can. Extend your arms straight from your shoulders towards the ceiling.
   Progression: Bring your feet away from the body. The further your feet are from you, the more challenging this exercise will be. If your spine leaves the floor, your feet are too far out.
2. Start the motion in the head by bringing your chin towards your chest.
3. Take 4 counts and continue the rolling motion through the spine; feel each vertebra leave the floor one at a time.
   Modification: Use the arms to assist your abdominals by pressing the elbows into the floor or walking the hands up the back of the thighs.
4. Fully erect the spine to sit tall. Lift chin up from chest.
5. Lower the chin towards the chest.
6. Hinge the upper body away from the thighs.
7. Take 4 counts and begin the roll down motion; allowing one vertebra at a time to lower onto the floor. Repeat at this pace 5-10 times.
8. Start the motion in the head by bringing your chin towards your chest.
9. Take 2 counts and continue the rolling motion through the spine; feel each vertebra leave the floor one at a time.
10. Fully erect the spine to sit tall; lift the chin from the chest.
11. Lower the chin towards the chest.
12. Hinge the upper body away from the thighs.
13. Take 2 counts and begin the roll down motion; allowing one vertebra at a time to lower onto the floor. Repeat at this pace 5-10 times.

   Rest and repeat the series 2-3 more times.

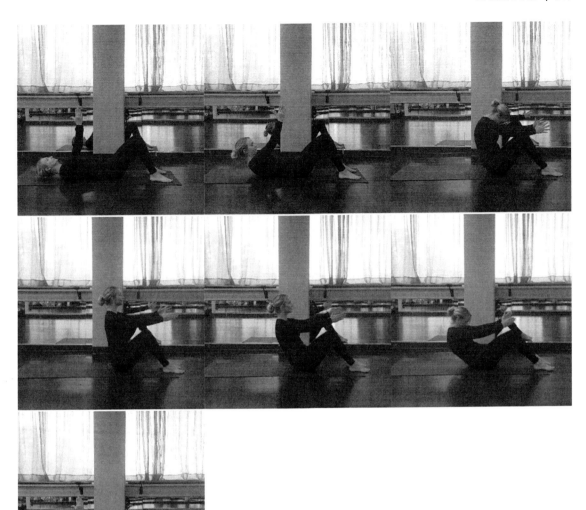

Roll-Up Notes:

-Make sure you keep your arms straight in front of the shoulders. The arms might want to swing back and forth to have momentum help you up and down.

-Don't forget to breathe! Inhale on the way up and exhale on the way down.

-Articulate through the spine on the way up and on the way down. Feel one vertebra at a time leave/return to the floor.

*PUSH-UPS:

1. On the floor, place your hands a little wider than your shoulders. Bring your knees back past your hips, not under them. Engage abdominals to support the spine.
    Progression: Attempt push-ups with your knees lifted off of the floor.
    Modification: Push-ups can be done at an angle on a bathroom or kitchen countertop.
2. Slowly bend the elbow to lower the chest towards the floor. Take 3 counts to lower and then lift in 1 count to return to starting position. Three counts down, 1 count up. Repeat 5-10 times.
3. Repeat the movement taking single counts down and up. Repeat as many times as you are able while keeping proper form. *Keep track of the number of repetitions you complete for your "Mile Marker."

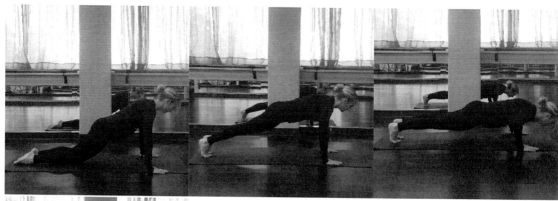

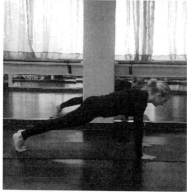

Push-up Notes:

-Be cautious not to drop your head towards the floor. Remember, your head is an extension of the neck which is an extension of the spine.

-Move in your pain-free range of motion. Whatever your joints allow you to accomplish.

-Pictures are in the progression form.

FROG LEG LIFTS:

1. Laying on your stomach, open your legs wider than your hips. Flex your feet, lift your feet from the floor, and press the heels together. Stack your hands on the floor and place your forehead on top of them.
2. Start the series by simply pressing the heels together and feeling the glutes, inner thighs, and hamstrings engage. Hold for 3 seconds.
3. Slightly release then repeat for 5-10 times.
4. Press the heels together. Taking 2 counts, use the glutes and lower back to lift the thighs from the floor.
5. Take 2 counts to slowly lower the legs back to the floor. Repeat 5-10 times.
6. Take 1 count to lift the legs.
7. Take 1 count to lower legs to the floor. Repeat 5-10 times.

   Repeat the series 2-3 times.

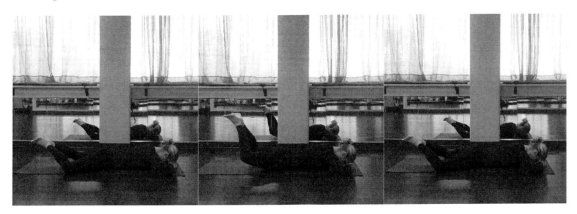

Frog Leg Lift Notes:

-If you are unable to lift the thighs from the floor, don't get discouraged. Keep trying and one day you will feel the air under your legs and celebrate!

-Keep the heels pressed together the whole time you are lifting the legs.

-Keep your abdominals engaged to help the hip bones from pressing too hard into the floor.

Fantastic job! Remember to cool down.

Week Four – Day Four

Isaiah 26: 3-4

> *"You will keep in perfect peace those whose minds are steadfast because they trust in you. Trust in the Lord forever, for the Lord, the Lord himself, is the Rock eternal."*

Steadfast. Unwavering. Constant. I hear these words and I think of characteristics of the Lord. They are, but in this passage, they describe how we are called to act. Insert gut check here! We should loyally keep our focus, hope, and trust in the Lord always. When we do so, we can expect God to give us a "perfect peace."

This week we are reading about how we are never alone; Jesus is always with us. And while we take rest in that fact, I'm confident there have been times you have felt alone - I most certainly have. Almost everyone I have spoken to on this subject has gone through a time when they didn't feel the Lord's presence in their life. We can re-read the verse above to know that when we don't feel Jesus, it doesn't mean He's not there. It could be because of our focus. Are you steadfast in your personal time with the Lord? Are you unwavering in your faith? Are you constantly searching for God's will in your life? When we are, there will be no denying the Lord's presence in our daily lives.

Jesus is with you always! During times of doubt, take inventory of your daily walk. I have learned that when I'm not feeling the Lord's comfort, it is because I am not seeking it properly.

Before moving on to today's fitness routine, think about what "perfect peace" means to you. Doesn't it sound absolutely amazing? What distractions are keeping you from achieving the peace you are meant to have through Jesus Christ?

DAY FOUR FITNESS ROUTINE

Please refer to Page xv for your warm up.

HIGH KNEES:

1. Standing with your ankles directly under your hips, bring your arms overhead. *Modification: Place your hands on your hips and omit arm movement during this series to alleviate any shoulder discomfort.*

2. Lift the right knee to hip height (or however high you can) and simultaneously lower the arms to bring the hands to the thigh.
3. Lower the foot to the floor and return arms overhead.
4. Lift the left knee to hip height while bringing the hands to the thigh.
5. Lower the leg and lift the arms back overhead. Repeat 10-20 times on each side moving at a challenging yet comfortable pace.
   Progression: Speed up the pace to involve a cardio aspect to this exercise.
6. Lift the right knee to hip height and twist the upper body to the right and bring both arms to the outside of the thigh.
7. Lower the leg, return to center, and bring the arms back up.
8. Lift the left knee and rotate the torso and bring the arms to the outside of the leg.
9. Lower the leg, return to center, and simultaneously bring the arms back up. Repeat 10-20 times on each side moving at the same challenging yet comfortable pace.

Repeat series 2-3 times.

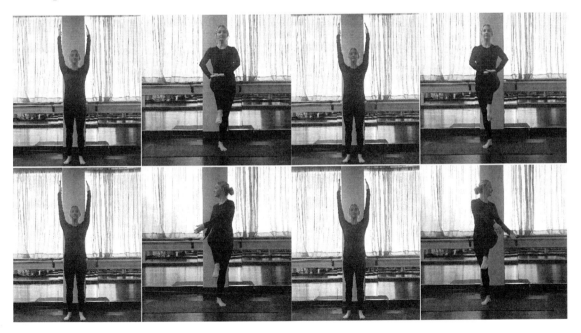

High Knee Notes:
-Challenge yourself to raise your heartrate during this exercise.

-During the twisting motions, keep abdominals tightly engaged to support the spinal movement.

*TRICEP PUSH-UPS:

1. Starting on all fours, place your hands directly under the shoulders with the fingers pointing forward. Bring your knees back past your hips. Engage the core so the spine does not dip towards the floor. Your neck is long.
   Progression: Lift the knees from the floor into a full push-up position.
2. Taking 3 counts, bend at the elbows allowing the arms to brush the sides of your body as your torso lowers towards the floor.
3. Take a single count to extend the arms to return to starting position. Repeat 4-6 times.
4. Reverse the counts. Take 1 count to lower the body and 3 counts to extend at the elbow to raise the body. Repeat 4-6 times.
5. Continue the same motion, taking 1 count down and 1 count to come up. Repeat as many times as you can while keeping proper form.

   Repeat series 1-3 times.

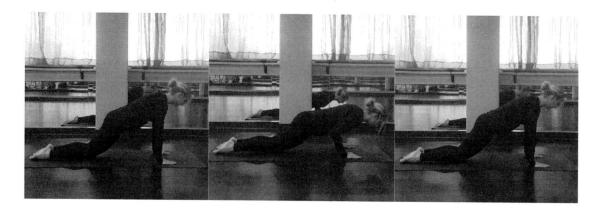

Tricep Push-up Notes:

*-*Due to the difficulty level of this exercise, the number of repetitions you are able to complete is your "Mile Marker."*

-Do not drop your head towards the floor.

-Keep the abdominals engaged to support the spine.

-Tell yourself to squeeze your ribs with your elbows. This will help you keep the arms close to the body.

-Allow the elbows to bend in such a way that they are "pointing" in the direction of your toes.

"D" LEG LIFTS:

1. Lay on your back with your arms by your sides. Bring your legs to table top and imprint your spine onto the floor. Contract the abdominals to roll the hips up towards the ribcage and press the spine down into the floor. Slightly extend your legs towards the ceiling.
2. Picture two capital "D's" back-to-back and trace them with your toes. They can be as big or as small as you like. Trace down the straight line, circle the legs out then up to the top of the "D." Repeat 5-10 times.
3. Reverse your motion; circle out then down to the bottom of the "D" then trace the straight line up. Repeat 5-10 times.

Repeat series 2-3 times.

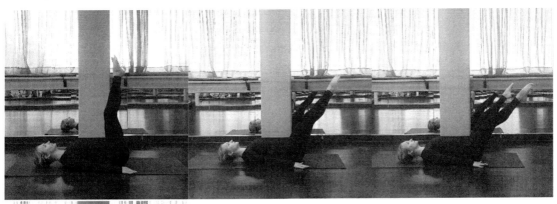

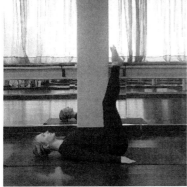

"D" Leg Lift Notes:

-If you would like support for your lower back, place your hands under your tailbone.

-Keep the spine imprinted on the floor during the entire series. If the back wants to come up from the floor, don't lower the legs as far. Keep the abdominals tightly contracted.

-If tightness in your hips occurs, bend your knees and shorten your range of motion.

BIRD-DOG GLUTE SERIES:

1. Begin on all fours with your hands under your shoulders and your knees under your hips. Contract the abdominals to lengthen the spine.
   Modification: For wrist discomfort, place elbows on the floor under the shoulders.
2. Slightly shift your weight to the left and lift the right knee to a hover over the floor. Flex the right foot.
3. Take 2 counts to lift the leg behind.
4. Take 2 counts to lower back under the hip. Repeat 10-15 times.
5. Take 1 count to lift the leg behind.
6. Take 1 count to lower the leg back down. Repeat 15-20 times.
7. Lift your leg behind you to your highest comfortable point. Contract the glute muscle to lift the leg an inch.
8. Slightly release the contraction to lower it an inch. Repeat this small pulsing motion about 30 times.
9. Rest and repeat on the left side.

   Repeat series 2-3 times.

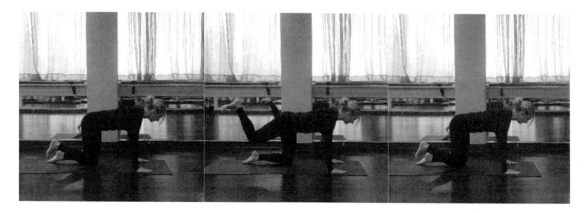

Bird-Dog Glute Series Notes:

- Only lift the leg up as high as you can without causing spinal movement towards the floor. Think of your back as a table top and don't let it move.

-You should feel engagement in your upper body and the stabilizing leg as they are working hard to balance and stabilize.

Great work today! Remember to stretch.

Week Four – Day Five

1 Chronicles 16:11

> *"Look to the Lord and his strength; seek his face always."*

Once again, the Bible is telling us to be active in our relationship with God. We must "look" to and "seek" Him daily. As Matthew 7:7 tells us, when we seek Him, we will find Him. In your times of weakness, when it comes to your health or anything for that matter, seek His strength to help you overcome temptations and hurdles. You will find it and can use it to master your situation.

As we look to the Lord and His strength, the Bible tells us to "seek his face". To do so, we must know what we're looking for. Have you ever met someone for the first time out in public? Years ago, I went through the experience of purchasing a used coffee table online. To make sure I was safely meeting the right person, we exchanged information. I knew what she looked like, what car she drove, and where she would be in the parking lot where we were meeting. She knew the same things about me. Without us knowing about each other, we could have put ourselves in a dangerous situation.

The same is true in our search for a love relationship with the Lord. We cannot send God an email and wait for His response to learn about Him. We must put in the time and effort to have a strong personal relationship with Him. Without knowing God personally, we put ourselves in danger when we go seeking security and answers to life's questions. To seek the Lord's face simply means to seek to know Him personally and we can do that by reading the Bible, meditating on His word, and listening for His gentle whispers.

Before preforming today's exercises, please re-read the Bible verse above. Do you know God? Do you know Him well enough to determine when you are face-to-face with His presence in your life? If not, why not?

DAY FIVE FITNESS ROUTINE

If needed, please refer to Page xv for you warm up.

*BICYCLE OBLIQUE CRUNCHES:

1. Lay on your back and bring both legs to table top position. Spread out your fingertips, cradle the back of your head, and bring the elbows away from the face. Lift your head and shoulder blades from the floor. Imprint your spine onto the floor.
2. Extend your right leg to the ceiling and lower it to a comfortable level where the spine is still in contact with the floor.
   Modification: Keep both legs bent with feet flat on the floor.
3. Rotate the upper body bringing the right shoulder towards the left knee. Hold for a count of 4.
4. Switch sides. Return the right leg to table top and extend the left leg in front. Rotate the upper body bringing the left shoulder towards the right knee. Hold for a count of 4. Repeat at this pace 4-8 times on each side.
5. Continue the same movement holding the crunch for 2 counts on each side. Repeat 6-10 times on each side.
6. Continue the bicycle motion speeding up the crunch hold for 1 count on each side. Repeat 8-12 times on each side.
   *Progression: *Move through the bicycle motion as fast as you can while keeping good form. Continue the "cardio cycle" for as long as you can. Keep track of your time and use this progression as a "Mile Marker."*

Repeat series 1-3 times.

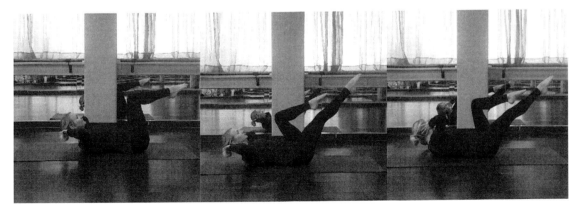

Bicycle Oblique Crunch Notes:

-Allow your elbows to be seen in your peripheral vision. If they are too wide, it can cause straining in the neck and shoulders. If the elbows are too close to the face, you're probably pulling on the neck causing unnecessary tension.

-If your hips start to feel tight, don't fully extend your legs.

-Make sure it's the shoulder and not the elbow that is aiming towards the knee. This will ensure proper oblique engagement.

-Allow the weight of your head to fully rest in your hands to minimize neck discomfort.

SPINAL EXTENSIONS:

1. Lay on your stomach with your hands stacked under your forehead and legs fully extended, reaching toward the wall behind you.
2. With hand remaining in contact with forehead and eye contact remaining on the floor below, slowly lift upper body from the floor to a challenging yet comfortable position. Lift chest up from the floor. If you aren't at that point yet, keep trying to reach this goal.
3. Return upper body to starting position. Repeat 10-15 times.
4. Slowly lift your straight legs from the floor. Make sure this motion is coming from the low back and the glute muscle (the rear end) and NOT the knees. You want to make sure the legs stay straight and reaching toward the wall behind you. Attempt to get some air under the thighs.
5. Return lower body to starting position. Repeat 10-15 times.
6. Lift the upper and lower body at the same time. Repeat 10-15 times.
   Modification: Alternate between upper and lower body.

   Repeat series 2-3 times.

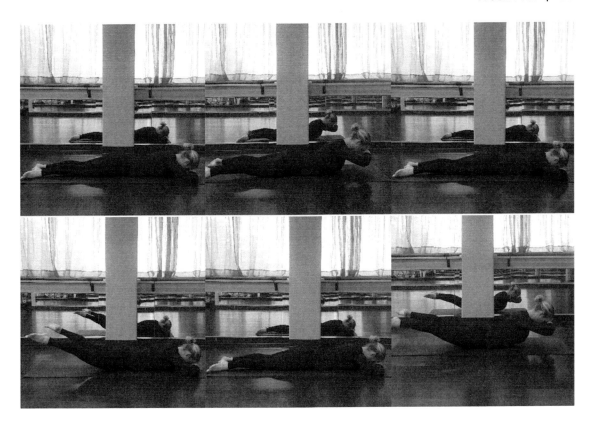

Spinal extension notes:

-*Make sure there is no movement from the neck. All movement should come from the low back and glutes.*

-*Continuously reach your legs long throughout the series. Toes should be pointed; calves, thighs, and glutes should be engaged.*

-*Engage abdominals to stay light in the hip bones. Pressing them into the floor can cause discomfort and takes effort away from the back extensors.*

PIKE TRICEP PUSH-UPS:

1. Start in a plank position. Lift the hips towards the ceiling. The shoulders will shift back. *Modification: In a knee plank position, omit the hips lifting towards the ceiling.*
2. Bend at the elbows, allowing them to move towards the feet and not out to the sides.
3. Extend the arms.
4. Return to plank position. Repeat 5-10 times.

Rest and repeat the series as many times as you can while keeping proper form.

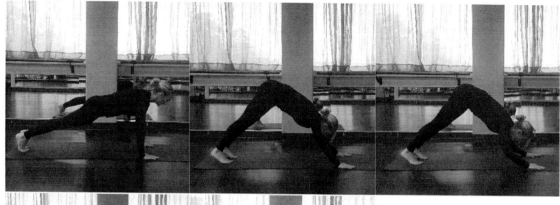

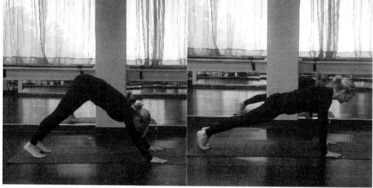

Pike Tricep Push-Ups:

-As the arms fatigue, the elbows will want to flare out to the sides. Keep your focus on the backwards movement of the arm bends.

-Be aware of dropping the head. Keep your eyes focused on the floor and not towards your feet.

BALANCE SERIES:

1. Stand with your heels together and your toes apart. Engage the core and stretch the spine tall towards the ceiling. Hands on your hips. If you know balance is not your strong suit, grab a chair or another prop to assist you.
2. Draw your right toes up the left leg. Open at the hip to the bring knee more towards the right. Engage your glutes.
   Progression: Take the toe away from the standing leg.
3. Slowly bring the knee in front of the hip. Moving at your own comfortable pace.
4. Slowly bring the knee back open to the starting position. Repeat 4-6 times.

5. Slowly extend and bend the leg. Repeat 4-6 times.
6. Moving at a faster pace if possible, continue to extend and bend the leg. Repeat the smaller movement 15-20 times.
7. Repeat series with left leg.

   Repeat series 1-2 times.

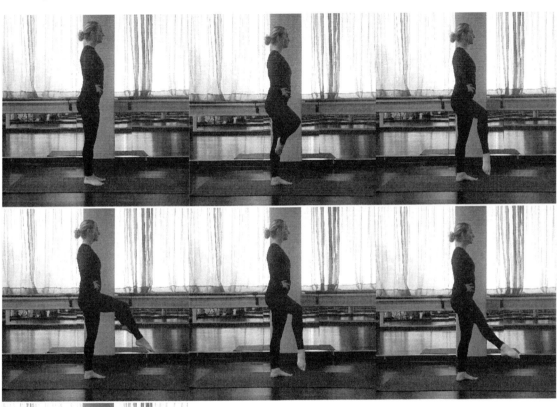

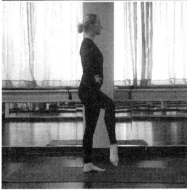

Balance Series Notes:

-If you need to take a quick break, go for it. Just get right back to it as quick as you can.

-Don't let the shoulders travel up towards the ears and create tension in the neck.

-Keep hips level.

-To help with balance, keep your eyes focused on a point on the floor that does not move.

Week Four – Day Six

1 Peter 5:6-11

"Humble yourselves, therefore, under God's mighty hand, that he may lift you up in due time. Cast all your anxiety on him because he cares for you. Be alert and of sober mind. Your enemy the devil prowls around like a roaring lion looking for someone to devour. Resist him, standing firm in the faith, because you know that the family of believers throughout the world is undergoing the same kind of sufferings. And the God of all grace, who called you to his eternal glory in Christ, after you have suffered a little while, will himself restore you and make you strong, firm and steadfast. To him be the power for ever and ever. Amen."

Today is the last day of the *BOW* program and I cannot think of a better verse to end with. What a great reminder of so many things:

1. Jesus cares for you.
2. You can give him all of your worries, doubts, and fears.
3. Satan is out to get you.
4. Stay strong in your faith.
5. You are not alone.
6. There will be suffering in this life.
7. God will restore and make you better than ever.
8. Power and glory to the Lord forever.

As you continue your journey of loving God sacrificially with your body, practicing self-control and self-discipline, bestowing grace to yourself, and focusing all of these efforts to develop a stronger relationship with the Lord, remember that you are more than capable to thrive!

You will have setbacks and obstacles to overcome, and that is okay. You are human and all humans have limits. But do you know what is so fantastic? We serve a God that is limitless! Hallelujah! Stay firm and stay healthy so you may serve God stronger and longer.

May you continue to worship God with your heart, soul, and BODY!

DAY SIX FITNESS ROUTINE

Refer to Page xv for you warm up.

LEG LIFT SCISSORS:

1. Laying on your back, bring your legs one at a time to table top position.
2. Imprint the spine; roll the hips up towards the ribcage until the spine is fully on the floor. Engage the abdominals to the point of pressing the spine deeply into the floor.
3. Extend your legs to the ceiling and lower the legs forward. Your spine should still be pressed firmly down by the abdominals. (This is your full range of motion.)
   Modification: Bend at the knees to shorten the lever. If you need support for your low back, place your hands under your tailbone.
   Progression: Reach your arms towards the ceiling.
4. Return the legs back to the ceiling.
5. Take 4 counts to lower the right leg towards the floor. If your spine begins to come off of the floor, you've lowered too far.
6. Take 4 counts to return the leg over the hip.
7. Repeat on left side. Repeat at this pace 2-4 times on each side.
8. Take 2 counts to lower the right leg towards the floor.
9. Take 2 counts to return the leg towards the ceiling.
10. Repeat on left side. Repeat at this pace 2-4 times on each side.
11. Shortening your range of motion, take 1 count to lower the right leg towards the floor.
12. Take 1 count to return the leg over the hip.
13. Repeat on left side. Repeat at this pace 2-4 times on each side.

Repeat series 2-3 times.

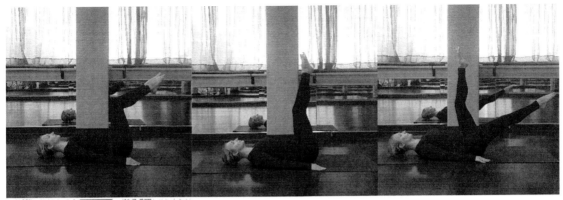

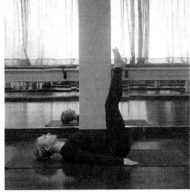

Leg Lift Scissor Notes:

-It is extremely easy to want to hold your breath during this exercise. Remember to breathe in through the nose and out through the mouth.

RUSSIAN TWISTS:

1. Sitting down with your knees bent in front of you and your feet flat on the floor, grab behind your thighs. Extended your arms and lean back. Engage the core. Lift the chin away from the chest.

   Progression: Lift both legs to table-top position and cross at the ankles.

2. Remove your hands from your legs and extend them straight in front of the shoulders.

   Modification: Keep hands behind the thighs to allow the arms to assist the abdominals.

3. Rotate the upper body to the right and tap the floor with the finger tips.

   Modification: If tapping the floor requires more of a twist than your back likes, omit the tap and keep the arms at shoulder height.

4. Lift the arms back to shoulder height and come back center.
5. Repeat on the left side.

   Repeat 10-15 times on each side.

6. Rest if needed. Repeat the series attempting to do an additional 5 more on each side.
7. Rest. Repeat the series and challenge yourself to do as many as you can while keeping proper form.

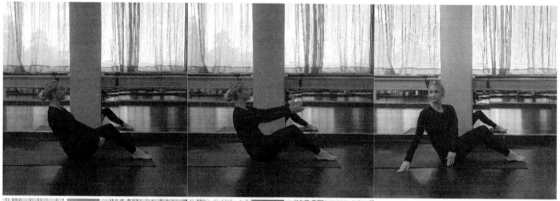

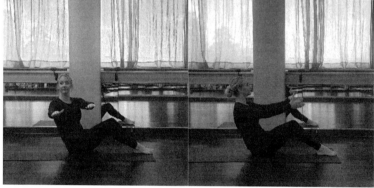

Russian Twist Notes:

-As you continue through this series, your abdominals may fatigue. If you need to, sit up tall and omit the leaning back to decrease the intensity.

-Make sure you aren't just moving the arms, but the entire upper body. Imagine you have a flashlight on your chest and you are scanning the room with the light.

DONKEY KICKS:

1. Begin on all fours with your hands under your shoulders and your knees under your hips. Engage the core by bringing the ribs and navel towards the spine in a baring down motion.
    Modification: Lower down to your elbows to alleviate wrist discomfort.
2. Drop your chin to your chest, roll the hips towards the ribcage, and round out the spine towards the ceiling. At the same time, bring your right knee towards your chest.
3. Carefully and at your own pace, lift the head to gaze up towards the ceiling, roll the hips back, and lower the navel towards the floor. Simultaneously, extend and lift the right leg behind you. Repeat 10-15 times.
4. Repeat on the left side.

    Repeat series 2-3 times.

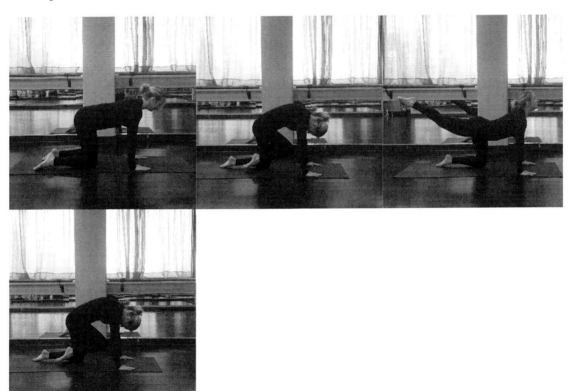

Donkey Kick Notes:

-Moving at your own comfortable pace is important in this exercise to protect your back.

-Make sure you have control of your leg as you lift it behind you. If you wildly kick it back, you could harm your lower back.

-As you lower and arch the spine towards the floor, keep abdominals engaged.

SIDELINE SERIES:

1. Lay on your right side with your right arm extended under the head. Stack your hips, knees, and ankles. Bring your legs in line with the rest of your body. Left hand on the floor in front of your chest to help with stability.
   Modification: Bend your bottom leg to increase support and stability.
2. Engage your core. You should feel it in your front, sides, and back.
3. Take 2 counts to lift your top leg towards the ceiling.
4. Take 2 counts to lower the leg back down. Repeat 5-7 times.
5. Take 1 count to lift your leg towards the ceiling.
6. Take 1 count to lower your leg down. Repeat 8-10 times.
7. Lift your leg half-way up and, from the hip, move your leg in a circular motion (about the size of a soccer ball). Repeat 5-7 times.
8. Reverse the circular motion. Repeat 5-7 times.

   Repeat on the right side 2-3 times.

9. Repeat the series on the left side.

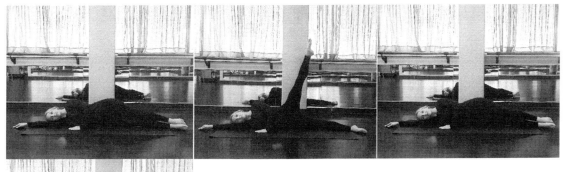

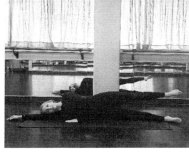

Sideline Series Notes:

-Pay attention to your top supporting arm. The goal is for your abdominals to do most of the stabilizing with the top arm assisting. If the top arm is getting tired, you are probably depending on it too much for stabilization.

-Work in your pain-free range of motion.

-When working in the circular motion, close your eyes and picture tracing the soccer ball sized circle. This visualization is a great distraction from the exercise itself.

Job well done! Enjoy your cool down on Page xix.

CONGRATULATIONS ON COMPLETING *A BODY OF WORSHIP*!

It has been an honor to go on this journey with you these last four weeks. It is my hope and prayer that the principals we have discussed throughout this program stay with you as you grow and develop healthier habits in every aspect of your life.

Going forward, remember what Jeremiah 29:11 says… "For I know the plans I have for you," declares the Lord, "plans to prosper you and not to harm you, plans to give you hope and a future." God is with you every step of the way and wants nothing but the best for you.

I would love to hear from you and hear all about your BOW experience. I am here for you and will continue to encourage you through social media @abodyofworship. We are in this together!